CORNWALL COUNTY LIBRARY

3 8009 03420 2561

D0346094

Food

Comments on *Food Allergies: Enjoying Life with a Severe Food Allergy* from readers:

'This book is packed with detailed and useful information.'
Sarah Campbell, Homoeopath (and mother of three with eczema)

'. . . essential reading for any allergy sufferer or their friends and family.'
Reviewer from London, featured on the Amazon website

'It is a really useful book and full of sense.'
Hazel Gowland, Allergy Action

'This is the most comprehensive help for food allergy sufferers that I have ever read.'
Maureen Jenkins, Trustee and Member of the Health Advisory Panel of Allergy UK,and Allergy Nurse Consultant, Sussex Allergy Service

'. . . and this edition is really excellent'
Michelle Berriedale-Johnson, Editor of *Foods Matter*

REVIEWS OF THE FIRST EDITION

'The author suffers from food allergy, but is also a state registered dietician with professional expertise on the subject. The result is a really detailed and useful book on the medical science of food allergy but, perhaps more importantly, the day-to-day practicalities of diagnosis and management of food allergy. The text is clear and comprehensive, and there is detailed description of the different types of special diets. Eating in or eating out: the author provides information that can be viewed as an oasis of accuracy on a topic about which much inaccuracy exists. Particularly useful is also the large section with addresses and web-sites for those wishing more information.'
Practice Nurse Journal

'Required reading for those with food allergies.'
David Reading, OBE, Director, The Anaphylaxis Campaign

'Tanya Wright has amalgamated her personal experience of severe food allergy with her expertise as a specialist dietitian to produce this unsurpassed guide to living with food allergy. I challenge anyone to find a question about the subject of food allergy that is unanswered in this wonderful book.'
Maureen Jenkins, Nurse Adviser and Coordinator of Training, British Allergy Foundation

'This excellent book will be a godsend for people who have food allergies, their carers and clinicians. I am often asked to recommend a single text which might help patients, carers and professionals to understand food allergy and the practical aspects of dealing with it. Tanya Wright's book would seem to be the perfect choice.'
Nursing Times

Food Allergies

Enjoying Life with a Severe Food Allergy

Second edition

Tanya Wright, BSc (Hons), RD

Registered Dietitian, working for Buckinghamshire Hospitals NHS Trust as Specialist Dietitian and Allergy Coordinator for adults and children attending the Allergy Clinic

Medical adviser: **Dr Joanne Clough** DM, FRCA, MRCP, FRCPCH

CLASS PUBLISHING · LONDON

Text © Tanya Wright 2001, 2007
© Class Publishing (London) Ltd 2001, 2007

All rights reserved. Without limiting the rights under copyright reserved above, no part of this publication may be reproduced, stored in or introduced into a retrieval system, or transmitted, in any form or by any means (electronic, mechanical, photocopying, recording or otherwise), without the prior written permission of the above publisher of this book.

Tanya Wright has asserted her right as set out in Sections 77 and 78 of the Copyright, Designs and Patents Act 1988 to be identified as the author of this work wherever it is published commercially and whenever any adaptation of this work is published or produced including any sound recordings or files made of or based upon this work.

Printing history
First published 2001
Second edition 2007

The information presented in this book is accurate and current to the best of the author's knowledge. The author and publisher, however, make no guarantee as to, and assume no responsibility for, the correctness, sufficiency or completeness of such information or recommendation. The reader is advised to consult a doctor regarding all aspects of individual health care.

The author and publishers welcome feedback from the users of this book. Please contact the publisher.

Class Publishing, Barb House, Barb Mews, London W6 7PA, UK
Telephone: (020) 7371 2119
Fax: (020) 7371 2878
Email: post@class.co.uk
Visit our website: www.class.co.uk

A CIP catalogue record for this book is available from the British Library

ISBN 13: 978 1 85959 146 8
ISBN 10: 1 85959 146 9

10 9 8 7 6 5 4 3 2 1

Edited by Gillian Clarke

Designed and typeset by Martin Bristow

Index by Vicki Robinson

Printed and bound in Finland by WS Bookwell, Juva

Cornwall Library	
Askews	
	£19.99

Contents

ENJOYING FOOD

Foreword

by **David Reading,** OBE
Director, The Anaphylaxis Campaign

Food allergy has become big news during the last decade. Rarely does a week go by without a dramatic story appearing in the newspapers or on TV. Peanut allergy, in particular, has become a source of sensational news reports and often the reader is left in no doubt that allergies can be serious. On rare occasions they kill.

Yet the help available for the food-allergic patient is often appallingly inadequate. It depends to some extent on where you live. Many doctors in general practice or running allergy clinics provide a wealth of vital information and practical guidance. But all too often, patients emerge from their consultation feeling totally despondent and unprepared to face the challenges ahead. The burden that families face is often overwhelming, particularly if it is a child who has a potentially severe food allergy.

As a founder member of the Anaphylaxis Campaign – a national charity set up in 1994 to help people manage their allergies – I became aware from the outset of the huge gaps in information available. Every day, we receive urgent appeals for help: What can I do to educate my child's school? Can I trust food labels? What do the results of my allergy tests mean?

Thankfully, there are people around who have made it their business to investigate the problems of food allergy, identify solutions and pass on their knowledge to others. Tanya Wright, the author of this book, has lived with severe milk allergy for fourteen years, and during that time has encountered most of the pitfalls. She has learned crucial lessons the hard way, and developed the message that it is perfectly possible to enjoy life with a severe food allergy so long as you are well equipped with information.

A huge amount of that information is presented in this book, making it an indispensable guide. Bon appetit!

Foreword

by **Maureen Jenkins**
*Trustee and Member of the Health Advisory Panel of Allergy UK,
and Allergy Nurse Consultant, Sussex Allergy Service*

Although true food allergy affects a minority of people, the incidence of food allergy is still rising. The severity varies between individuals but it has a daily impact on those affected and their families or carers, involving continual monitoring of all ingredients consumed. These are often 'hidden' or called by strange names. Most foods that cause potentially life-threatening reactions are those most commonly eaten or their components frequently used in food manufacture.

Allergy is difficult to understand and many people find it impossible to obtain specialist professional advice or diagnosis, causing anxiety and despair. Many resort to alternative therapies that may exacerbate their problems, but here Tanya Wright advises how to obtain a specialist referral.

This inspiring book eloquently explains, in everyday language, the mechanisms within the body that cause an allergic reaction and provides solutions to the numerous problems faced by people with food allergy. Although there are many books about food intolerance, very little has been produced to adequately help those with true food allergy. The author has amalgamated her personal experience of severe food allergy with her expertise as a specialist dietitian in this fantastic guide to living with food allergy.

This latest edition includes an update on the food allergen labelling laws. New allergens, such as lupin, are explained along with a comprehensive list of food families and potential cross-reactions. There is practical help with special diets and alternative foods, eating out and foreign travel, plus a large appendix with cross-referenced links, names and addresses of specialist food manufacturers and an extensive product update.

You will find current advice on managing anaphylaxis. Career and leisure choices and information about help agencies are all thoroughly covered. There is also guidance on prescribed and over-the-counter medicines that may contain allergens and comment on the possibility of state benefits.

This is the most comprehensive help for food allergy sufferers that I have ever read.

Author's note

The purpose of writing this book was to bring together both my professional and my personal experience of living with a severe food allergy. It is aimed at people with a severe food allergy and their families, and the healthcare workers helping them, to provide a useful resource as well as a source of comfort for those living with this condition.

Reading this book and using the relevant information should help you to *Enjoy Life with a Severe Food Allergy!*

Acknowledgements

We are very grateful to the many people who have helped in the development of this book. In particular, we thank:

Dr Joanne Clough, for allowing us to use some Glossary entries from her book *Allergies: Answers at your fingertips*

and for their reviews of the manuscript:

Marianne de Giorgio, mother of children with food allergies

Lorna Downing, mother in a family with food allergies

Hazel Gowland, food adviser to the Anaphylaxis Campaign, who also gave permission to use the food names translation chart

Maureen Jenkins, Allergy Nurse Consultant, Sussex Allergy Service

Arthur Ling, Managing Director of Plamil Foods

Dr Anna Moore, MBBS, DipNutritional Medicine, a GP with Special Interest in Nutrition

David Reading, OBE, Director of The Anaphylaxis Campaign

Hazel Rollins, CBE, Nutrition Nurse Specialist at Luton & Dunstable Hospital NHS Trust

Grieg Saunders, Product Manager at Provamel

Muriel Simmons, Chief Executive of Allergy UK

Isabel Skypala, Director of Rehabilitation and Therapies at the Royal Brompton & Harefield NHS Trust, and Specialist Allergy Dietitian

Christopher Swire, of Fayrefield Foods Ltd

Victoria Wick, Product Manager at Matthews Foods

About the author

Tanya Wright is a registered dietitian specialising in the diagnosis and management of food allergy and intolerance. She works within the Buckinghamshire Hospitals NHS Trust with both adults and children. Her role there is to co-ordinate the allergy service, to write the patient information diet sheets and factsheets, to manage her clinical dietetic workload and to organise and deliver the food challenge service. She provides information and resources on allergy for other healthcare professionals within and outside the Trust.

She is also author of two colour recipe books: *Allergy-free Food* (Hamlyn 2002) and milk-free recipes for infants (Cow & Gate 2006). She has also contributed to the book *Latex Intolerance* (CRC Press 2005).

Tanya regularly lectures both at national conferences and to students to Masters level. She writes articles and recipes for special diet food companies, formula milk companies, magazines, newspapers, websites and supermarket chains, and is a regular consultant to the food industry, to allergy support associations and to other health professionals. Tanya is on the committee of several organisations, including the British Dietetic Association food allergy and intolerance specialist group (FAISG) where she contributes to the production of position papers and is the resources officer.

She is due to complete her Masters in 'The Mechanisms and Management of Allergic Disease' at Southampton University in 2007.

About the medical adviser

Jo Clough trained as a paediatrician, specialising in allergic disease. She is a Fellow of the Royal College of Physicians. Jo worked as a paediatric physician specialising in asthma and allergic diseases and was a Senior Lecturer at the University of Southampton. She now works as a medical adviser and is the author of *Allergies: Answers at your fingertips* (also published by Class).

Introduction

The fact that you are reading this book suggests that either you or someone in your family (or perhaps both) has an allergy or intolerance a food or foods. At a relatively minor level, eating the 'wrong' food can bring you out in a rash (hives). At an extreme level, eating even a minute amount of a trigger food can cause a very serious reaction – anaphylaxis. (Anaphylaxis can also be caused by a bee or wasp sting or a drug or latex products, among other things, but in this book we will be talking only about food allergy.)

Anaphylaxis can be life-threatening, and people at risk of this severe reaction should carry adrenaline with them to use in such an emergency. It seems to have become more common in recent years, but in fact affects less than 1% of the population.

A number of well-publicised deaths caused by food-induced anaphylaxis have highlighted the fact that preventive measures as well as prompt treatment have an essential part to play in living with this life-threatening condition. Most cases are triggered by food eaten outside the home. In fact, most of the deaths due to food-induced anaphylaxis have resulted from food eaten in restaurants, cafés and other busy commercial eating-places.

Media coverage and pressure groups such as the Anaphylaxis Campaign have greatly increased awareness of the practical problems of living with the threat of anaphylaxis. Food manufacturers and retailers and the food and catering industries are making many positive changes to their practices and labelling to minimise the risks to susceptible people ingesting foods to which they are allergic.

The information in this book will complement the work that is taking place by enabling you to be more proactive in preventing severe reactions to food. If you do experience an allergic reaction, having a plan of action and all the necessary treatment to hand is the foundation of successful management. Even if you are not at risk of the most severe form of allergy, the information here will help you to live a normal life despite having to avoid certain foods or ingredients.

Terms that might be unfamiliar are explained at their first mention. They are also included in the Glossary at the back of the book.

Background

1
Food Allergy

WHAT IS ALLERGY?

An allergy is an inappropriate and harmful response of the body's defence mechanisms to substances that are normally harmless. Allergic reactions involve the immune system, which protects us from infections by viruses, bacteria and parasites. When a potentially harmful attacker, such as the measles virus or a staphylococcus bacterium, invades our body, the many different parts of the immune system work together, signalling to one another using chemical messengers, to surround and kill the attacker before serious damage is done. The first time the body encounters a new type of germ, it will be several days before the infection is overcome. However, the immune system retains a memory of the attacker, so that future infections are dealt with promptly and efficiently. This memory is in the form of *antibodies*, which are small proteins that are tailor-made for each attacker. There are several different types of antibody, and the main ones involved in fighting infections are immunoglobulin G (IgG), immunoglobulin A (IgA), immunoglobulin M (IgM) and immunoglobulin E (IgE).

In people who develop allergies, the immune system works perfectly well against infectious organisms. In addition, though, it has a tendency to react to normally harmless substances as if they were attackers. When this happens, the immune system becomes *sensitised* to the substance – it mistakenly identifies the substance as a hostile factor and, by producing antibodies against it, programmes the body to react whenever it is encountered. Substances that cause this reaction are known as *allergens*, which are almost always protein molecules. When the body encounters an allergen, even in tiny amounts, large quantities of allergy antibodies (immunoglobulin E, or IgE) are made, which react with the allergen to set off a series of events called the *allergic reaction*. This process involves many different parts of the immune system, co-ordinated by chemical messengers released by the white blood cells.

Most of the damage to the body's tissues that occurs during an allergic reaction is a result of the release of the chemicals from a type of cell called the *mast cell*. (Mast cells are one of the cells that make up the immune system and are found in many different tissues of the body. They are particularly common in the airways of the lung, in the bowel wall, and in the eyes, nose and throat.) These chemicals are stored inside the mast cell in tiny packages, or granules. When an allergen reacts with the IgE antibodies on the surface of the mast cell, these granules are released. The chemicals in them have a number of effects, including the enlargement of small blood vessels, increased leakiness of the blood vessel walls, the contraction of the muscle in the bowel wall and lung airways, and the increased secretion of mucus. These changes lead to the redness, tenderness and swelling commonly known as inflammation.

This allergic inflammation has different effects in different parts of the body. In the lungs it causes coughing and wheezing – the symptoms of asthma. In the nose it may cause runniness and block-age – the symptoms of rhinitis or hay-fever. In the bowel it may cause colicky pain and diarrhoea, or, in the mouth, itching and tingling – the symptoms of food allergy. Sometimes the allergic reaction involves the skin, leading to itching and rashes.

WHO CAN DEVELOP ALLERGIES?

Anyone can develop allergies but individuals whose parents or siblings have allergic disease have a greater tendency than others to develop an allergy at some time in their lives. The most common allergic diseases are asthma, eczema and hay-fever. The tendency to develop an allergy, known as *atopy* (from the Greek 'atopia', meaning 'out of place'), seems therefore to be inherited. Atopic individuals are much more likely to develop allergic disease if they are exposed to certain environmental factors or *triggers*. (Allergy prevention is discussed in Chapter 11.)

HOW COMMON IS ALLERGY?

The number of people affected by allergy has increased dramatically in recent decades. Allergies now affect one-third of the population in the affluent countries of the industrialised world. In the UK one person in three has suffered from eczema by the age of 3½ and one child in eight is currently treated for asthma. It is predicted that, as Third World countries develop, a similar pattern will emerge.

The World Health Organization has labelled allergy 'the number one environmental disease'.

Food allergy

Although as many as 20% of the population believe they are allergic to one or more foods, it is estimated that more like 2–3% of adults and 6–8% of children have *true* food allergy. By the time children are 5 years of age, around 85% of these grow out of egg allergy, and 95% grow out of the most common childhood food allergies – milk allergy.

The 'Allergic March'

'Allergic march' is a medical term used to describe the way allergy develops with age. It reflects the fact that children who suffer from food allergy often go on to develop other allergic conditions later in life: eczema, asthma and rhinitis (hay-fever). For this reason research into preventing allergy from developing in the first place is really important (see Chapter 11).

WHY ARE ALLERGIES INCREASING?

It is thought that a number of environmental factors may increase people's susceptibility to allergy. They include modern housing, the Western diet, family size and the over-use of antibiotics.

Housing

As a result of double-glazing, good insulation and efficient heating systems, the humidity and temperature of our homes and work/ social environments have risen to levels that encourage high numbers of house dust mites, whose faecal droppings contain an allergen. This, plus an increase in the use of soft furnishings (carpets, curtains, cushions) in which the house dust mite thrives and the growing popularity of pets (which produce allergens), means an increase in allergen levels. The effect is increased because people now tend to spend more time indoors.

Diet

There is some evidence to indicate that changes in our diet also play a part. Whereas several decades ago most food was fresh, nowadays much of it is processed and contains many additives. Moreover, processed foods contain fewer natural antioxidants and vitamins, which are abundant in fresh fruit and vegetables, and which are thought to protect against a number of conditions – including allergic diseases.

The age at which certain foods are consumed may also be important. See also the box at the end of Chapter 11, 'Allergy Prevention'.

Family size and childhood infections

Children from smaller families seem to be more likely to develop an allergy. This is thought to be because they are exposed to fewer viral infections in early life than children in larger families, and therefore don't have the opportunity to build up an immunity. This applies especially to those who have not attended nursery or playgroup. Frequent infections in early life promote a switch to the non-allergic response as opposed to the allergic response, which makes it much less likely that an individual will develop an allergic condition in later life.

Antibiotics

The increasing use of antibiotics in early life (and their inclusion in foodstuffs via animal feed) may alter the balance of the 'friendly' bacteria found on the skin and in the bowel. This may, in turn, increase the risk of developing allergic diseases.

All these theories are backed by scientific evidence but the full picture remains unclear.

FOOD HYPERSENSITIVITY

'Food hypersensitivity' is an umbrella term for any unpleasant, reproducible reaction to food. This hypersensitivity is divided into food allergy and non-allergic food hypersensitivity (Figure 1.1).

Non-allergic food hypersensitivity covers:

- metabolic defects such as lactose intolerance,
- pharmacological reactions such as the effects of caffeine and alcohol,
- biological contamination such as food poisoning,
- toxic reactions such as scromboid food poisoning,
- and other food intolerances and aversions.

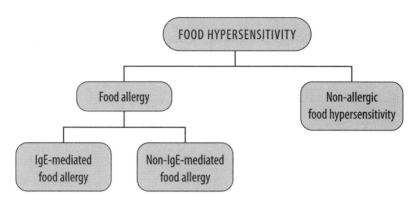

Figure 1.1 Types of food hypersensitivity

Food allergy (allergic food hypersensitivity) is split into reactions that are IgE and non-IgE mediated.

IgE-mediated food allergy

IgE-mediated reactions are associated with immediate symptoms that include itching, red skin, hives, angioedema and, in its most severe form, anaphylaxis, a potentially life-threatening reaction. Anaphylaxis is the most extreme reaction of a food allergy, and is discussed in Chapter 4.

The foods most commonly implicated in these reactions in the UK are cow's milk, egg, peanuts, nuts and soya in children, and fish, shellfish, peanuts, nuts and wheat in adults. Across Europe and the rest of the world the common foods differ.

Non-IgE-mediated food allergy

Non-IgE-mediated reactions are usually symptoms related to the gut and skin, such as eczema, vomiting, diarrhoea and constipation.

The most common 'provoking' foods include milk, egg, wheat, soya, chocolate, additives and artificial colours.

This book focuses on information to help people with reactions caused by IgE-mediated reactions, particularly anaphylaxis. However, it is also relevant to people with other types of food hypersensitivity, particularly in the 'enjoying food' and 'enjoying life' sections.

What happens during an IgE-mediated allergic reaction?

An allergic reaction to food can cause a range of symptoms in a number of different parts of the body:

- swelling of the lips, tongue and face (angioedema),
- itchy 'nettle' rash (urticaria/hives),
- wheezing and shortness of breath,
- runny nose and inflamed eyes (rhino-conjunctivitis),
- swelling of the voicebox (larynx),
- colicky abdominal pain, diarrhoea, nausea and vomiting,
- life-threatening collapse with shock (anaphylaxis),

as well as flushing, palpitations, feelings of anxiety and faintness.

All these reactions are caused by immune responses involving IgE antibodies. They occur very quickly after the allergen has been ingested – usually within minutes. Occasionally, symptoms can come on after a delay of a few hours.

TREATMENT

How severe reactions are treated is discussed in Chapter 4. The treatment of less severe reactions will depend on the symptoms, and may involve avoiding a specific food (or foods), or taking antihistamines or any of a variety of therapies specific to the individual's symptoms. Exclusion diets are useful in identifying food intolerances and less severe food allergies. They are discussed in Chapter 8 ('The Dietitian's Role').

SUMMARY

You should now understand more about what happens during an allergic reaction. Later in this book you will find out about the different types of food allergies and their management.

2
Food Allergy Tests

Allergy testing carried out by your GP or at an allergy clinic may help to identify which substances you may be allergic to. But the appropriate tests can be chosen only when the details of your medical history have been considered. Unfortunately, no allergy test will predict the nature and severity of your reactions in the future.

WHAT TO DO IF YOU THINK YOU HAVE A FOOD ALLERGY

You may suspect you have a food allergy, for a number of reasons, and you may also feel that you know what the offending food is. However, to be sure of the exact nature of the allergy and for the correct treatment to be prescribed, the allergens should be identified by your doctor using safe and accurate methods.

Before you keep your appointment with your GP or the allergy specialist, note down as much information as possible about your symptoms. You can use the following checklist as a guide to the sort of information to keep:

- Your symptoms: what, where, when, for how long?
- The exact circumstances leading to the symptoms; for example:
  - what had you eaten?
  - how long after you ate it did symptoms begin?
  - where had you eaten it?
  - were there other foods around at the time?
  - who had prepared the food?
- Your own and your family's history of atopic disease (asthma, eczema, hay-fever, food allergies, anaphylaxis).
- Foods you think may have caused the symptoms.
- Other factors that might have caused the reaction.
- Frequency of the reactions.
- Details of past reactions.
- Details of medication taken following a severe reaction.
- Any exercise before or after eating.

Keeping a record of these facts will help the doctor to diagnose your problem and, if it is due to allergy, to identify the allergens. Even if you know what is causing your reaction, it is still important to go through this process for confirmation to ensure that an allergy is indeed the problem and, if so, to check for any cross-reactivity and to see if you are allergic to any other allergens. With cross-reactivity, two or more allergens induce similar reactions. The allergens may be from the same food group or from different food groups (see Chapter 12, 'Cross-reactivity and Food Families').

DIAGNOSIS OF A FOOD ALLERGY

Diagnosing a food allergy and identifying the offending foods is done largely on the basis of your medical history but may also require allergy testing. These tests should be performed and interpreted by a practitioner with the appropriate training and experience, because no test is 100% reliable. All results should be considered in relation to your history and symptoms.

A diagnosis of food allergy can be made if there is:

- a positive medical history (usually confirmed by a positive skin-prick test or RAST) (see below), *or*
- a positive medical history plus a positive response to a 'food challenge' in which neither you nor the person doing the testing knows what the food being tested actually is (a double-blind food challenge), *or*
- a positive medical history plus a positive objective response to 'open challenge' (i.e. both you and the person doing the testing know what foods you are being given).

Diagnosing yourself (self-diagnosis) is inadvisable. If, for example, you cut too many foods out of your diet without adequate nutritional replacement, you may become malnourished. For this reason it is essential to obtain recognised professional help when trying to detect food allergies. Once a food allergy has been diagnosed you may then be referred to a state registered dietitian, who will give you detailed advice on which foods to avoid and how to replace them with suitable alternatives so that you can maintain a nutritionally balanced diet (see Chapter 8, 'The Dietitian's Role').

TESTING FOR A SUSPECTED FOOD ALLERGY

Once a food allergy is suspected, one or more of the following tests may be done to confirm the diagnosis. Usually the simplest tests are done first.

Skin-prick test (SPT)

This is the most commonly used, fastest and easiest way to detect an allergy. The basis of a skin-prick test is that it demonstrates the presence of allergen-specific immunoglobulin E (IgE) attached to the skin's mast cells (see Chapter 1). It involves placing a liquid extract of the suspected allergen on the skin (usually the forearm) and pricking the skin through it so as to just puncture the skin, without drawing blood. If there is a positive reaction to the sample allergen, a small bump (called a weal) will come up, reaching its maximum size within 10–15 minutes. It looks quite like nettle rash and is likely to be red and itchy, and may have a flare (the skin immediately around the itchy lump may go red). The reaction disappears within an hour.

Fresh foods can be used in the skin-prick test: some people are allergic only to foods in their raw state, so prepared allergens are unsuitable.

Any number of allergens can be tested at a time, but it is important that only relevant (suspect) foods are tested. Each area of the skin that is being tested is marked with a pen, so that the reaction can be identified later. The amount of allergen introduced into the skin is so tiny that a serious reaction is extremely unlikely. In addition to the allergens to be tested, positive and negative 'controls' are used to ensure that the test is being performed correctly.

The **negative control** is a saline (salt water) solution, to which no response is expected. If there is a response, it may be that the skin is over-sensitive to pressure and that the response to the test is a 'false positive'. If this happens, the doctor will interpret the results with the utmost care, and may even decide that the whole test is invalid.

The **positive control** is a solution containing a standard concentration of histamine, to which everyone is expected to react. If there is no response to the positive control solution, it is possible that something is preventing the skin from reacting to the allergen. A number of drugs can do this, including all antihistamine preparations, some antidepressants, some cough mixtures and, under certain conditions, preparations that contain steroids. These medications should, if possible, be stopped one week – or even, in some cases, up to one month – before the skin testing. (If you are waiting to see the GP or allergy specialist for an initial appointment, it may be useful to contact them to find out when you need to stop your medication.)

It is possible to have an unexpectedly positive result to a skin-prick test that does not fit in with your medical history. There are several reasons why this might happen. For example:

- The food extract used in the test is not identical to the actual food that you eat.
- The allergen may be prepared differently from when it is used in food (e.g. raw rather than cooked).
- The testing site may have been contaminated with a substance to which you do react.
- The test has been administered improperly.

A *false negative result* might be obtained if:

- the IgE antibodies are located in the mucous membrane of the reaction site and not in the blood,
- the person being tested is on certain medications, as mentioned earlier;
- the extract used is of poor quality or is out of date.

These problems are relatively uncommon, and the skin-prick test is a useful tool in the diagnosis of a food allergy, especially as the results are visible and fairly immediate. It is, however, important that a doctor experienced in this field interprets the test results.

Blood test – radio-allergosorbent test (RAST)
For this test (now also called the specific IgE test), a small sample of your blood will be taken from a vein in your arm and sent to a hospital laboratory for testing. The results – which are usually available in 7 to 14 days – are a measure of the amount of IgE produced in response to individual allergens. Results are graded according to the strength of the reaction. Blood tests are not affected by antihistamines, so they can be used with people who cannot stop taking them.

RASTs are relatively expensive, so should be used in conjunction with other tests such as skin-prick testing. Examples of when this blood test is indicated include:

- in people with extensive skin lesions (e.g. eczema), in whom interpreting skin-prick tests is difficult,
- in people who have had a severe allergic reaction, in whom skin-prick testing may be dangerous,
- if solutions of the relevant allergen are not available,
- in people who are unable to stop taking their antihistamine medication,
- where skin-prick tests are unavailable.

The results of RAST tests are sometimes classified from 0 (negative) rising to 4 or 6 (extremely high) – the scale used will depend on the hospital. For example:

Class	Level of sensitivity to the tested allergen
0	Negative
1	Low
2	Moderate
3	High
4	Extremely high

In most hospitals this grading has been replaced with unit values instead, which is more accurate.

As with skin-prick tests, it is possible to get false negative and false positive results with RAST tests. For this reason and because the range of allergens available for testing is not fully comprehensive, the results of these tests should not be viewed alone, without knowledge of the person's medical history and food and symptom diaries (see below).

Food challenge test

The two types of 'food challenge' used most commonly are:

- **Open food challenge** You are given increasing quantities of the food to which it is thought you are allergic and your symptoms are noted. In this test both you and the person administering the food know what it is.
- **Double-blind placebo-controlled food challenge** Both the food in question and a harmless dummy (the placebo) are given

in random order, often hidden in capsules, so that neither you nor the doctor knows which food (if any) is being taken. This is important because sometimes an unpleasant reaction to food can occur because of psychological associations; for example, if you have previously been very ill after eating seafood, just the sight of seafood might make you feel sick.

A food challenge may be offered when:

- there is uncertainty as to whether a food allergy exists,
- it is supected that an allergy has been outgrown,
- confirmation of a suspected allergy is required,
- a food is to be taken for the first time (e.g. when a food has been avoided for many years because of a history of allergy in the family),
- skin-prick test results are negative,
- RAST results are negative or greatly diminished.

This test will be performed in hospital – either in the outpatient department or in a ward – by a person trained in the management of severe allergic reactions. (This is because there is a small chance that a severe reaction might occur.)

Because of the time and resources required to undertake food challenges, they are available in only some hospitals and so the waiting list can be long.

The food/symptom diary

A food/symptom diary can be very useful in determining which foods cause an allergic reaction. Every time you have a reaction, note down everything you have eaten and drunk, giving the date and time, and then record the time and details of any symptoms you experience. (Remember to keep the labels of any prepacked foods you consume.) The information gained will give valuable clues to aid your diagnosis. Figure 2.1 shows you how to draw up a chart to fill in.

Date	Time	Food/Drink consumed	Time	Symptoms

Figure 2.1 Example of a food and symptom diary

Dietary manipulation

Once food allergens have been identified successfully, it is necessary to completely avoid the offending food(s) and any derivatives of these foods. To do this successfully usually requires the help of a dietitian (see Chapter 8), who will advise on avoiding food(s) and replacing them with substitutes of similar nutritional quality.

ALTERNATIVE DIAGNOSTIC THERAPIES

Complementary medicine practitioners and their skills have a lot to offer and they can provide very effective therapies for *some* conditions. However, there are many 'alternative' allergy tests on offer that are *not* regarded by conventional practitioners to be relevant and are considered to have no place in the diagnosis of true allergy. These include kinesiology, hair analysis, iridology, pulse test, sublingual provocation test, urine test, sweat test, radionics and vega testing, to name a few. They may be offered through supermarkets, health-food shops, health farms, newspapers, the *Yellow Pages* and glossy magazines.

The drawbacks of having such tests are:

- the method of testing is inappropriate,
- the resulting diagnosis may be inaccurate,
- inappropriate and unbalanced diets may be recommended,
- it is often suggested that a large number of foods are avoided for an indefinite period of time, with little or no adequate dietary review,
- failure to recognise and treat a genuine disease,
- they are often undertaken by unqualified staff,
- the creation of fictitious disease entities.

Any of these can lead to malnutrition and disturbed growth in children, unintentional weight loss, food phobias, frustration and anger when things do not improve, disruption of one's lifestyle and a poor quality of life. The only valid tests for food allergy are skin-prick tests, RAST and food challenge, and possibly patch tests.

FOLLOWING THE DIAGNOSIS OF A FOOD ALLERGY

If you are diagnosed as having a food allergy you should be referred to a dietitian, who will give you advice about the foods and ingredients that you can eat safely and devise a management plan. For a severe food allergy this will involve:

- total exclusion of the offending food from your diet,
- replacement of excluded foods with others of similar nutritional value,
- making sure that you fully understand the new diet and are able to follow it,
- arranging for follow-up appointments from time to time as long as you need them, to deal with any problems or questions.

If your child has been diagnosed as having a severe food allergy, it will be important to make sure that friends, playmates and school staff fully understand it. Liaising with your child's school is dealt with in Chapter 6 ('Food Allergy and Going to School').

The role of the dietitian is discussed more fully in Chapter 8.

TESTING FOR LATEX ALLERGY

Allergy to certain foods may be related to an allergy to latex ('cross-reactivity', discussed in Chapter 12). A suspected latex allergy can be tested by a number of methods, including a patch test, a skin-prick test or a RAST.

A positive result to any of these tests means that efforts must be made to avoid any contact with latex; individual advice should be sought. If you are in hospital or at the dentist, it is essential that you ask for non-latex examination gloves to be used. This is particularly important if the procedure is to happen under a general anaesthetic, as you will not be awake to remind the staff at the last minute when the gloves come out! Latex is also found in blood pressure cuffs, theatre table covers, medical equipment, etc., etc.

REFERRAL TO AN ALLERGY SPECIALIST

If you have, or suspect that you have, an allergy, the first port of call is usually your general practitioner (GP). If your GP feels that further investigation is required, you may be referred to a specialist in allergies. Allergy specialists are usually part of an NHS hospital-based allergy clinic, and their services can be accessed only by referral from either a GP or a hospital doctor. Self-referral is not an option in the UK.

Obtaining a referral from the GP is not always straightforward. Sometimes people feel that they should have been referred to an allergy clinic but their GP did not sanction it. This may be because the GP had the necessary skills required to give the advice. Most allergy services in the UK are provided by GPs, paediatricians (children's doctors), chest or respiratory physicians (e.g. for asthma), dermatologists (for skin problems, such as eczema) and doctors specialising in ear, nose and throat (ENT) conditions (such as rhinitis). Although these provide a valuable service, there is a need for more specialists trained in all aspects of allergy.

Another possible reason for non-referral might be that the GP was unaware of the availability of this service and how to locate it.

GPs who wish to locate their nearest NHS allergy clinic can consult the British Society for Allergy and Clinical Immunology (BSACI) website (see Appendix 2), which provides information on allergy services in the UK. Allergy is a very broad subject and the services provided by allergy clinics can vary enormously, so this site is designed to provide GPs and referring doctors with detailed information about each clinic, so that they can refer appropriately.

The doctors in NHS allergy clinics are usually members of the BSACI, which recommends the standards of care in such clinics. They will be aware of the Code of Good Allergy Practice, outlined in the *Standards of Care for Providers of Allergy Services within the NHS*, supported by the BSACI.

There are too few NHS allergy clinics in the UK to cope with the increasing number of people with severe allergies, which is why there are often long waiting lists. The allergy clinics that do exist are not evenly spread geographically, which may mean people having to travel long distances.

A study published in 1999 by the BSACI (the professional body for doctors working in allergy) reported that the UK has only five NHS clinics offering a full-time multi-disciplinary allergy service, with a further 115 providing only part-time services. These figures equate to only one full-time allergist for every 2.1 million population. There have been various campaigns to raise awareness of the inadequate provision.

The Department of Health's 2006 report *A Review of Services for Allergy* recommends the following action to be taken over the next few years in order to improve allergy services:

- local commissioners of health care to establish levels of need for allergy services,
- work towards additional training places for allergy specialists,
- develop with the National Institute for Health and Clinical Excellence (NICE) guidelines for allergy work, and work with the Royal Colleges on guidance for referral of patients and care pathways.

3
Will My Allergy Improve over Time?

People with a severe food allergy often ask about the likelihood of growing out of it or, if this is not possible, if there are alternatives to living with it, such as an allergy vaccine or a medical treatment. Although there is no drug treatment for food allergies, this chapter discusses the possibilities.

IMMUNOTHERAPY (DESENSITISATION)

Immunotherapy (also known as 'desensitisation') is a well-established treatment for certain allergies – for example, for pollen and bee sting – but *not* for foods. Starting with a minute dose, increasing doses of an allergen are administered until you can tolerate exposure to it without developing major symptoms. Immunotherapy to cat and grass is available in only a small number of UK centres, and then only for people with a single sensitivity for whom conventional treatment has failed or who are in high-risk occupations.

VACCINE

A lot of research work is investigating the possibility of vaccine therapies for food allergy. There are two types: 'non-specific' therapies, which reduce allergic symptoms to everything to which a person is allergic; and 'specific' therapies, which reduce symptoms to individual allergens to which the therapy is directed (e.g. Brazil nut allergy). Researchers are evaluating these two approaches to blocking food allergy reactions.

There has been much media hype about curing allergies with some form of allergy vaccine or drugs. In reality there are no such treatments currently available; however, vaccines are being trialled in several countries so there is hope for the future.

GROWING OUT OF IT

It is difficult to say whether someone will outgrow an allergy – at present we just don't know. However, there are some reports of outgrown nut allergies recurring. A possible explanation for this is that nuts were not eaten for long periods, which reduced tolerance. This suggests that, once an allergy is outgrown, the food should be a regular part of the diet. Research in the area is ongoing.

Children often outgrow allergies. Around 85% outgrow egg allergy and 95% outgrow milk allergy by the age of 5 years. Peanut and nut allergies are outgrown less often: some research has found that this may occur in 10–20%. As the child gets older, so the likelihood of this happening diminishes.

If you develop your allergy (or allergies) in adulthood, you are much less likely to outgrow it; but it is still possible.

Because allergies can be outgrown, an allergy review is recommended, particularly for children. Because egg and milk allergies are often outgrown, they are often tested for on a yearly basis in children under 5.

If you have not had a reaction for a number of years or think you have had inadvertent exposure to the food but no reaction, retesting is recommended. You should, however, continue to avoid all foods you have previously been avoiding until you have been advised otherwise at your allergy clinic. The specialist may offer skin-prick testing, a blood test, a food challenge or all three, depending on your clinical history.

If your allergy has been outgrown, it may be that you will no longer need your 'rescue medications' such as antihistamines and adrenaline. However, continue to carry them at all times until you have been advised otherwise.

4
Anaphylaxis

The word *phylaxis* is the Greek for 'protection', so *anaphylaxis* is the opposite to this. Anaphylaxis is the most severe form of allergic reaction. It is a medical emergency characterised by symptoms including shortness of breath, low blood pressure and collapse of the circulatory system that carries blood to the various organs. In extreme cases it is potentially life-threatening.

Although there is a wide range of symptoms that can occur in anaphylaxis, not all of them will be experienced on each occasion.

WHAT ARE THE CAUSES OF ANAPHYLAXIS?

Anaphylaxis, or an anaphylactic reaction, can have any of several causes, outlined below.

Certain foods Any food can cause anaphylaxis but the most likely culprits are nuts, peanuts, sesame seeds, fish, shellfish, cow's milk and eggs.

Exercise-induced anaphylaxis This usually arises only after eating a particular food, generally just before or just after exercise, although there may be a delay in some people. This type of anaphylaxis is therefore known as *food-dependent exercise-induced anaphylaxis*. Some susceptible people may be able to tolerate exercise alone or to eat a certain food with only a mild reaction or no reaction at all. However, exercise shortly before or after ingesting this food causes an allergic reaction. Finding out which food is having this effect may require allergy tests, and referral to an allergy clinic is essential for diagnosis and management.

Idiopathic Anaphylaxis that has no known cause, even after extensive testing, is known as idiopathic anaphylaxis.

Insect stings Every year in the UK there are between two and nine deaths from bee and wasp stings; hornets are another common cause of insect allergy. The risk of being stung can be minimised by taking precautions as outlined in the factsheet produced by the

Anaphylaxis Campaign (address in Appendix 1) or ask your specialist or GP.

Latex Gloves, condoms, balloons, elastic bands, rubber-soled shoes and many more items that are made from natural rubber latex can provoke a life-threatening allergic reaction. Latex allergy can also be associated with an allergy to certain foods; this 'cross-reactivity' is discussed in Chapter 12.

Medicines In susceptible individuals some medicines can cause anaphylaxis. Common examples are drugs containing salicylate (e.g. aspirin) and certain anaesthetics, but most drugs have the potential to cause an allergic reaction and are, in fact, the most common cause of anaphylaxis.

AT WHAT AGE CAN ANAPHYLAXIS START?

Anaphylaxis can start at any age. There are no rules, except that it is more likely to occur in an atopic person – someone who has inherited the susceptibility to allergy from a first-degree relative (parent).

WHAT ACTUALLY HAPPENS IN THE BODY?

When a susceptible person comes into contact with an allergen that causes an anaphylactic reaction to occur, that allergen becomes bound to the surface of the mast cells (see Chapter 1). The binding of the allergen to the surface of the mast cell causes it to release a number of different chemicals, or mediators, which have a profound effect on the organs of the body. In the skin they cause leakiness and relaxation of the small blood vessels, leading to flushing, swelling and characteristic rashes (urticaria and angioedema). In the lung they cause muscle spasm and narrowing of the airways, which become blocked and filled with mucus. In the gut there is also muscle spasm and leakiness of the blood vessels, causing colic and diarrhoea. The coronary arteries, which supply blood to the heart muscle, go into spasm, and damage to the muscle can occur. The veins collecting blood from the other organs of the body lose their tone and become larger and leaky, no longer doing their job properly. The blood pressure falls and the blood supply to all the major organs is compromised.

WHAT ARE THE SYMPTOMS?

The symptoms of anaphylaxis can vary in both severity and the speed with which they happen (speed of onset), even in the same person. Any of the following symptoms may occur:

- tingling of the lips or in the mouth,
- flushing of the skin or a generalised rash,
- swelling of the lips, mouth, face or throat, or hands and feet,
- nasal congestion,
- sweating and/or dizziness,
- difficulty in swallowing or speaking,
- abdominal cramps, nausea, vomiting and diarrhoea,
- wheezy chest,
- feeling of faintness and deep anxiety,
- weakness,
- collapse,
- loss of consciousness.

WHAT FACTORS INCREASE THE SEVERITY AND SPEED OF AN ALLERGIC REACTION?

It is thought that certain factors can increase the severity and speed of an allergic reaction. They are:

- poor general state of health,
- alcohol,
- exercise,
- ingesting a larger amount of allergen,
- stress,
- poorly controlled asthma.

WHAT IS THE TREATMENT?

Prompt treatment of anaphylaxis is essential and may be life-saving. Although histamine preparations may be used in the early stages of an allergic reaction, the mainstay of treatment is an injection of adrenaline (also called epinephrine). It is a very safe drug, which must be given as early in a reaction as possible. If prescribed, an asthma-relieving inhaler can be given as well.

It is also helpful if oxygen is given once medical help is available.

Antihistamines

Antihistamine medication is often used as the first line of treatment for the relief of a mild to moderate allergic reaction. The symptoms are caused by the chemical histamine, which is produced during the end-stages of an allergic reaction. Antihistamines work by blocking the action of this chemical, which thus reduces the symptoms of redness, itching, mucosal swelling (e.g. swelling tongue), excess secretions (e.g. runny nose) and allergic skin rashes.

You can buy certain antihistamines 'over the counter' (without a prescription), but there are many different types, so it is essential that you discuss with your pharmacist or your GP or allergy specialist the most appropriate choice for you. This is particularly important if you are taking any other medication. You should also get advice about when to take the antihistamine. Remember that, if the symptoms get worse, you *must* proceed to adrenaline (see below).

Side-effects of antihistamines

Modern antihistamines (e.g. acrivastine, cetirizine, loratadine) have very few side-effects. Be aware, though, that some of the older antihistamines can make you feel drowsy and affect your ability to operate machinery and to drive. At present there is no legislation governing the use of medicines when undertaking these tasks, but it is your responsibility not to do so if you have symptoms or side-effects that could affect your judgement. (This is also the case for some other medications and alcohol.)

Other side-effects associated with the use of certain antihistamines

In 1990 and 1992 the Medicines Control Agency (part of the Department of Health) issued safety warnings that terfenadine and astemizole could, in certain circumstances, be associated with the development of abnormal heart rhythms. The effect is rare and was found only in people who exceeded the manufacturer's daily dose or were taking other drugs that interacted with the histamine. Nevertheless, terfenadine and astemizole have been withdrawn from use.

Adrenaline

Adrenaline (epinephrine) in its natural form is a stress hormone that is produced in your body by the adrenal glands. Adrenaline causes the 'fight or flight' reaction, which prepares your body for any stressful activity by speeding up your heart and increasing the flow of blood to your muscles.

The medical form of adrenaline is given by injection during a severe allergic reaction in order to aid the reversal of the life-threatening symptoms that are associated with anaphylaxis.

Remember *always* to go to your nearest Accident & Emergency Department if you have an anaphylactic reaction, even if you feel better after using the adrenaline, because its actions are short-lived (see below). You may also have a secondary, delayed reaction or complications, so you need medical attention to ensure that all is well or to deal with any problems.

How does adrenaline work?

In anaphylactic shock, the blood vessels leak, the airways (bronchial) tissues swell and the blood pressure drops, causing suffocation and collapse. Adrenaline acts within seconds to constrict blood vessels, to relax muscles in the lungs and to stimulate the heart beat. This results in improved breathing, reduced swelling and improved circulation.

The EpiPen and Anapen are the most usual ways to inject adrenaline. They are available as a pre-loaded syringe that administers a single predetermined dose of life-saving adrenaline into the thigh. In most cases the beneficial effects are felt within seconds.

Anyone who is at risk of having an anaphylactic reaction is usually advised to carry two adrenaline injector pens. This is because the duration of action of adrenaline is short (about 10 minutes) – if there is a delay in obtaining medical attention the effects of the initial dose of adrenaline may wear off and a second dose may be required.

Larger adults may also need more than one because the amount of adrenaline required is related to body weight.

If you need to carry an EpiPen or Anapen, do practise often with the trainer pen so that you are completely familiar with it. Also practise on an orange with an expired pen – this feels quite different from the trainer pen.

EpiPen The EpiPen has a spring-loaded, concealed needle that delivers the dose when the pen is jabbed against the outer thigh and then held in place for 10 seconds. Available only on prescription, it comes in two forms: EpiPen and EpiPen Junior.

- The *EpiPen* delivers a dose of 0.3mg of adrenaline for adults and children weighing over 30kg.

- The *EpiPen Junior* delivers a dose of 0.15mg for children 15–30kg.

Babies and children under 15kg will be prescribed adrenaline in the most appropriate form.

EpiPen trainer pens are available to practise with. As well as having one at home, it is a good idea to have one in the child's pre-school or school setting, so that those responsible for administering it can familiarise themselves with it. In addition, the EpiPen website (details under Alk-Abelló in Appendix 1) has a video clip showing how to use it correctly.

Instructions for administering the EpiPen and EpiPen Junior are given on the side of the injector:

1. pull off grey safety cap,
2. hold EpiPen near outer thigh with black tip pointing towards outer thigh,
3. swing arm away from thigh, then jab firmly into outer thigh – through clothing if necessary – until the pen clicks,
4. hold in place for 10 seconds,
5. remove pen and massage thigh.

Anapen The Anapen is another preloaded adrenaline syringe that carries a single measured dose of adrenaline. It has a mechanism whereby, on pressing a firing button, a spring-activated plunger pushes the needle into the thigh muscle. It is then held in place for 10 seconds.

- The *Anapen* delivers 0.3mg adrenaline for adults and children over 30kg.
- The *Anapen Junior* delivers 0.15mg for children weighing 15–30kg.

Lincoln Medical, the distributors of all the Anapen products, will supply the *Anapen trainer pens* on request, for a small fee. The Anapen and Anapen Junior can be obtained only with a prescription.

To use the Anapen:

1. remove the black needle cap,
2. remove black safety cap from firing button,
3. hold Anapen against outer thigh and press red firing button – through clothing if necessary,
4. hold in position for 10 seconds, allowing the full dose of adrenaline to be injected.

Care of your prescribed adrenaline

- Adrenaline should not be stored above 25°C. It should never be refrigerated or frozen. For suggestions on how to keep your adrenaline at the correct temperature in hot weather, see Chapter 16 ('Holidays and travelling').
- Adrenaline easily degrades when exposed to direct sunlight. If this happens, it may not work as effectively. For this reason, it should be kept in its outer case until it is required. You can buy special bags to carry your adrenaline and rescue medication (e.g. from Yellow Cross or Kidsaware; contact details in Appendix 1) or you can use an old glasses case or pencil case.
- The adrenaline should be a colourless liquid. If it becomes discoloured or contains a precipitate (solid matter), you will need to replace it. You can check the liquid through the observation window. If you have any concerns, take it to your pharmacist who will check it for you.
- Remember to replace your adrenaline injector by or even before it reaches its expiry date. (Take expired ones to the chemist or pharmacy for safe disposal.)
- Your prescribed adrenaline and rescue medication should be carried at all times.
- As with all medication, store it out of reach of children.
- Make sure that young people who do use medication know how to use it and look after it.

You should check your adrenaline injectors on a regular basis to ensure that they are in-date and in good condition (colourless and without precipitates). However, in an emergency, provided that it is in good condition, the use of out-of-date adrenaline is better than no adrenaline at all..

Side-effects of adrenaline

The most common side- (unwanted) effects of adrenaline are trembling, palpitations (an awareness of the heart beat), sweating, a fast heart beat, nausea, dizziness and a feeling of anxiety or tension. Despite these effects, don't be afraid to use this life-saving medication. They are the normal effects of adrenaline, which soon wear off. In fact, some people don't even notice them when adrenaline is administered in the recommended dose.

WHICH MEDICATION – AND WHEN?

When to take, or give, medication is understandably a cause of great concern. The most common question asked by people who have experienced moderate to severe allergic reactions is: 'At what stage of an allergic reaction should the prescribed antihistamine and adrenaline be taken?' There is, unfortunately, no way of knowing in advance how severe a reaction will be, but a good general guide is:

- For symptoms such as a rash, sneezing or an itchy throat, where there is no shortness of breath or feeling faint, initially use the antihistamine.
- If the reaction develops to include symptoms such as shortness of breath or feeling faint, adrenaline should be administered without delay.
- If the reaction includes breathing difficulties or feeling faint from the very beginning, miss out the antihistamines and give the adrenaline immediately.

If adrenaline is necessary, an ambulance should also be called immediately, because the beneficial effects of adrenaline may be short-lived and further treatment may be necessary.

Table 4.1 Quick guide to 'which medication?'

Medication	Indications	Symptoms
Antihistamine Syrup or tablets or **Bronchodilator (blue) inhaler**	Mild reactions	Itchy hives Rash Wheeze
Adrenaline injection given via: EpiPen/EpiPen Junior or Anapen/Anapen Junior	Severe reactions	Swelling tongue Short of breath Feeling faint Floppy Losing consciousness
Steroid tablets/syrup (e.g. prednisolone)	After an anaphylactic reaction that has been successfully treated with adrenaline	Acute symptoms are resolved

Two things can threaten life in anaphylaxis:

- Difficulty breathing, when the air passages become restricted – due either to swelling in the throat and upper airways or to narrowing of the small airways as in asthma.
- Circulatory collapse, leading to inadequate supplies of oxygen to the tissues of the body.

If treatment with adrenaline is not given until the reaction becomes this severe, it is less likely to be successful.

If you are in doubt whether the reaction has progressed enough to warrant the adrenaline, it is best to go ahead and use it. The risk of not having the adrenaline when it is needed far outweighs the negligible risk of taking or giving the adrenaline unnecessarily.

Table 4.1 is a quick guide on which medication to use, and when.

TREATMENT WHEN TAKING OTHER MEDICATION

If you have some other condition such as high blood pressure or an abnormal heart rhythm, or are on certain other medication, you should seek medical advice about the safety of using adrenaline.

Beta-blockers and ACE inhibitors (used by people with high blood pressure) may make adrenaline relatively ineffective. Other treatments are available and these should be discussed with your GP or allergy specialist without delay.

Asthma

People with asthma are at greater risk of developing a severe or even potentially fatal anaphylactic reaction. Therefore, if you are in any doubt as to whether your symptoms of wheezing and breathlessness are due to straightforward asthma or are part of a severe allergic reaction, you should administer adrenaline without delay and take your bronchodilator (blue) inhaler if you have one.

Anaphylaxis mistaken

Anaphylaxis can be mistaken for conditions that have similar symptoms, such as hyperventilation, panic attacks, alcohol intoxication and low blood sugar (hypoglycaemia). This is an important reason for wearing some sort of medical identification jewellery that will tell others of your condition if you are unable to do so yourself (see Chapter 5, 'Your Anaphylaxis Contingency Plan').

Fatal anaphylaxis

Fatal anaphylaxis is rare but, owing to a lot of media coverage over the past few years, deaths due to food allergy seem to be more common than they are.

The fact that you are reading this chapter means you are trying to find out all you can about anaphylaxis, so that you understand it and know what to do if it does occur. You are more likely to ensure that you wear emergency identification and more likely to check food labels and methods of food preparation. All of this not only reduces the risks of a reaction occurring but also increases the likelihood of your receiving prompt and correct treatment if it is required.

The importance of information and understanding about anaphylaxis for people with an allergy and for their friends, relatives and guardians should not be underestimated.

Anaphylaxis at school

This subject is discussed in Chapter 6.

MANAGEMENT OF A SEVERE ATTACK

Have a written action plan in place and follow it.

Anyone who receives emergency adrenaline should be taken to the hospital accident and emergency (A&E) department immediately. Dial 999 and inform the controller that the person is suffering from anaphylaxis. If symptoms persist, or improve and then recur, a second dose of adrenaline may be required.

It is always important to seek emergency medical help even if adrenaline has been administered. The duration of action of an adrenaline injection may be as short as 10 minutes and, if symptoms recur, further treatment such as antihistamines and corticosteroids (steroids) might be needed. It will also be necessary for the person to be observed for a suitable period of time to make sure that recovery is complete.

Once in hospital other medication may be given, including oxygen, fluids, antihistamines and corticosteroids.

Even with adequate treatment with adrenaline, repeat attacks have been known to occur up to eight hours later. For this reason observation in an A&E department is recommended for up to eight hours following life-threatening anaphylaxis, and four hours for milder reactions.

SPEEDING UP THE TREATMENT IN AN EMERGENCY

- Always wear medical identification.
- Have an action plan for treatment that is:
  - accessible,
  - easy to read,
  - easy to understand,
  - easy to implement,
  - up to date,
  - in the correct language if you are abroad (see Chapter 16, 'Holidays and Travelling').
- Carry at least two syringes of adrenaline at all times.
- Carry an antihistamine at all times.
- Be confident about when to take the antihistamine and when adrenaline is required.
- Tell others about your allergy and action plan for treatment.
- Have access to a mobile phone and charger at all times for emergency use.
- Ensure that an ambulance is called even if you have administered the adrenaline and feel better. The person calling the ambulance should always state that you are having an anaphylactic reaction, as this is a medical emergency where time is of the essence.
- Get more information if you are unsure of any of the above.

What to expect in the A&E department

The precise treatment you receive when you reach hospital will be specific to the severity of the reaction and your symptoms. Table 4.2 is meant purely as a general guide.

HOW CAN YOU PREVENT FURTHER REACTIONS?

The only way to prevent a further attack is to avoid the substance that caused it. If you are unsure about the cause, it is essential to seek advice from your GP, who may refer you to an allergy clinic (see Chapters 2 and 3).

Table 4.2 What to expect in the A&E department

Action	Reason
You are lain down	In case of fainting because of the drop in blood pressure during anaphylaxis
A small plastic tube (intravenous cannula) is immediately inserted into a vein, usually in your hand or arm, and a 'drip' set up	To gain access before the veins shut down, so that medication and fluid can be administered
Adrenaline from a syringe (not an auto-injector) is given via the cannula – if not already given, or a second dose is required	Because the action of adrenaline reverses the symptoms of anaphylaxis
An oxygen mask is placed on your face	To increase the level of oxygen in your blood; the level drops during anaphylaxis
You are attached to a machine that monitors your blood pressure	To check that your blood pressure is returning to normal levels
You may be given hydrocortisone or other corticosteroids via the cannula	To reduce the swelling associated with anaphylaxis
Treatment continues as above until you are stable	To stabilise your blood pressure
You will be kept in A&E for observation: about 4 hours for a mild reaction, 8 hours for a severe reaction or overnight if required	In case a secondary reaction occurs that requires treatment, and for monitoring purposes
You may be given hydrocortisone tablets to take at home for 1 to 3 days	To prevent the likelihood of a delayed or secondary reaction
Letter written to your GP	To keep the GP informed and so that another adrenaline auto-injector can be prescribed if it has been used. For referral to an allergy clinic if required.

THE ANAPHYLAXIS CAMPAIGN

The Anaphylaxis Campaign is a charity that provides evidence-based advice, information and support to susceptible people and their families about all aspects of anaphylaxis.

The charity also campaigns for better allergy services in the UK and highlights anaphylaxis issues to the government bodies that make decisions on food policy. The aim of this is to improve food manufacturing, labelling and preparation practices to help reduce the risks to susceptible people of consuming a substance that may trigger an allergic reaction. It is advisable for all people who are at risk of anaphylaxis and their families to join the Anaphylaxis Campaign (address in Appendix 1).

THE PHARMACY AND THE 'LITTLE RED BOOK'

Increasingly we look to the pharmacist for help and guidance. The Code of Ethics of the Royal Pharmaceutical Society of Great Britain states that 'pharmacists must do everything reasonably possible to help a person in need of emergency medicines or treatment'. In 1999, a guide was written for community pharmacists to use as a reference. Called *Emergency First Aid: professional standards*, and often known as the 'Little Red Book', it outlines the most appropriate treatment of medical situations that are likely to arise. It gives guidance on the action to be taken in life-threatening situations – including anaphylaxis – when it is believed that a pharmacist would be justified in administering certain medicines without a doctor's prescription.

Many pharmacy/chemist shops in the UK have a copy of this book, which is certainly reassuring if you have a severe allergic reaction in the High Street and need help while you are waiting for the ambulance to arrive.

The booklet can be obtained from the Royal Pharmaceutical Society (contact details in Apendix 1).

FREQUENTLY ASKED QUESTIONS*

When and how should I carry my EpiPen?
It should be carried with you at all times – in a pocket or a handbag or in a protective case. Do not remove it from its outer yellow case until you need it.

Where should I store my supply of EpiPens?
EpiPen should be kept at room temperature and not refrigerated. If it is exposed to extreme heat or sunlight, the adrenaline will turn brown. Check that the adrenaline is clear by looking through the viewing window of the auto-injector.

Where do I inject the adrenaline?
EpiPen should be injected only into the outer thigh, through clothing if necessary. Do not inject EpiPen anywhere else. (Trainer EpiPens are available for teaching the injection technique.)

Can I use a second EpiPen?
Usually one pen is sufficient, but if symptoms do not improve or they get worse or return, a second EpiPen may be administered five minutes after the first one. EpiPens can now be prescribed as a two-pen pack.

Why is it important to seek medical attention immediately after using the EpiPen?
Further treatment and observation in hospital may be necessary because the symptoms of anaphylaxis might return.

How do I discard my adrenaline auto-injector after use?
Place the auto-injector back in the plastic case and give it to the emergency services, who will dispose of it safely.

What should I do with my out-of-date EpiPens?
When you go to collect your new EpiPens, give the out-of-date ones to the pharmacist, who will dispose of them safely.

* Although this box is about the EpiPen, the general comments also apply to the Anapen.

5
Your Anaphylaxis Contingency Plan

By taking all the precautions discussed in this book, you should rarely, if ever, have a severe reaction. Nevertheless, you may accidentally eat or drink something that you would normally avoid, so you should always have a contingency plan just in case. Also included in this chapter are some more general information and helpful hints.

EMERGENCY PACK

The emergency pack described below contains information and medication that may be required if you have a serious allergic reaction. It is recommended that you have access to this pack *at all times*.

Information card
This contains essential information about you and how to contact your next of kin (NOK) or some other person (ICE) – in case of emergency.

EMERGENCY MEDICAL INFORMATION

Name: Mrs A L Lergy
Address: 140 Adrenaline Close, London HE 1P
Tel: (H) 0123 456 789 (W) 0987 654 321
NOK/ICE: (Husband) Mr E C Zema
Tel: 0111 222 333 **Mobile:** 07988 777 666

Medical Information
Severe allergy to: Milk and dairy products
　　　　　　　Eggs

IN THE CASE OF A SEVERE ALLERGIC REACTION, *I REQUIRE ADRENALINE*
I carry adrenaline for emergency use. Please administer this in an emergency and then dial **999** for an ambulance.

Identification (ID)

Special medical identification is especially useful if you are unable to communicate your needs (you may be unconscious, breathless or unable to speak clearly). With this identification your medical condition can be diagnosed and the correct treatment given. The faster the diagnosis is made, the sooner the life-saving adrenaline can be given. (ID is discussed in more detail later in this chapter.)

Two adrenaline auto-injectors

It is recommended that you carry two adrenaline auto-injectors (EpiPen or Anapen). This is because, if the first one does not relieve the symptoms after five minutes, a second dose will be required.

Antihistamine

When the symptoms of a reaction start, you will not usually know if it will develop into full-blown anaphylaxis. For this reason it is useful to take an antihistamine (tablets or syrup), which is sometimes enough to stop the reaction developing any further.

Mobile phone

A mobile phone can be extremely useful to communicate quickly with those who may be able to help in an emergency. This includes alerting nearby friends/family and for calling an ambulance.

ACTION PLAN FOR USE IN SEVERE ANAPHYLAXIS

1. Remove the EpiPen/Anapen (adrenaline auto-injector) from the yellow tube.
2. Remove the grey safety cap.
3. Inject the adrenaline by jabbing the EpiPen/Anapen firmly against the thigh (instructions on the side of the autoinjector).
4. Call 999 for a paramedic ambulance, stating that it is for an anaphylactic reaction (severe allergy).
5. Give a second dose of adrenaline if the first one has not taken effect after 5 minutes.
6. While waiting for the ambulance, lie down with your feet raised.
7. When the ambulance arrives, make sure the paramedic is given your Emergency Pack, including the used autoinjector.

Action plan

The information cards in this emergency pack can be written with help from your GP or allergy specialist.

It is essential that you make up an emergency pack such as the one outlined above, and that friends and family know of its existence. If you have an anaphylactic reaction, the pack will make it possible for the correct procedures to be undertaken before paramedics arrive and take over. Precious seconds will be saved in administering life-saving medication. In anaphylaxis *time is of the essence*.

GENERAL PREPARATION

Below is a checklist for you to make sure that you are prepared in the event that you have an anaphylactic reaction.

MY EMERGENCY CHECKLIST

☐ I have made up an emergency pack.

☐ I have checked the contents of my emergency pack with my GP or allergy specialist.

☐ I keep a check on the 'use by' date of my antihistamines and adrenaline auto-injectors to ensure that they are always in date.

☐ If I use the adrenaline auto-injector(s), I always order replacement(s) immediately.

☐ I do not expose my adrenaline auto-injectors to extremes of temperature.

☐ I keep my friends, family and colleagues informed about my allergy and the contents of my emergency pack.

☐ My friends, family and colleagues have a 'role-play' practice from time to time (about every three months) of the procedures to be taken in an emergency, using the EpiPen or Anapen Trainer.

☐ If I have a mobile phone, I always keep it charged and have an in-car charger in case the batteries run flat when I am in my car.

☐ I have a visible note about my severe allergy on the dashboard of my car.

☐ I carry with me identification that explains about my severe allergy.

If you are able to tick all the boxes in the checklist, you can rest assured that you are doing all you can in preparation for an emergency – which, hopefully, will never happen.

IDENTIFICATION (ID)

Even with the best will in the world, accidents do happen. So it is essential that you are prepared for the possibility of an allergic reaction.

In a medical emergency it is not always possible to give details about your medical condition, so carrying identification is an easy way to inform members of the public and the medical profession about your allergy. This gives vital information about your condition, thereby assisting diagnosis and speeding up treatment so that critical seconds are not lost. The earlier the life-saving adrenaline is given, the greater the chance of a positive outcome.

Young children who are under constant supervision do not usually wear ID but this is an individual decision.

Types of ID

Jewellery
Identity jewellery generally comes in the form of a necklace, bracelet or watch. These are available from the following (contact details in Appendix 1):

Medic-Alert Foundation The Foundation has a selection of identification jewellery with an internationally recognised medical symbol, engraved with your medical condition and a phone number for the emergency services to call for all your details. There are Medic-Alert affiliates throughout the world. An initial fee is charged, plus an annual fee.

Medi-Tag This is similar to the Medic-Alert system. The jewellery available is similar, plus a watch.

SOS Talisman A necklace or bracelet with an internationally recognised medical symbol is unscrewed to access a 'concertina' of information inside. Details are filled in by the wearer.

ID jewellery can be expensive. If you are on a low income, you may be able to get financial help from a local charity. Contact the company that you are considering buying from and they will probably be able to offer further advice on this.

Clothing and accessories

Kidsaware (contact details in Appendix 1) produces 'awareness' clothing and accessories for babies and children with allergies.

Yellow Cross Company (contact details in Appendix 1) has a range of bags, ID tags and cards for children and adults.

Identity cards

These come as a card or laminated card, and can be obtained from many self-help organisations. If you have to complete the details yourself, it may be useful to get help from your GP or allergy specialist to ensure that the details and terminology are correct.

Badges

Some parents make or have made material, metal or plastic badges that announce their child's allergy such as 'Do not give me nuts' or 'I am allergic to eggs'. This can make some children feel special but others may feel the odd one out. Nevertheless, it is important to keep people informed about a child's allergy without making the child feel isolated or 'different'.

Tags

Local key cutters and engravers will often make up key rings or tags (or anything else you can suggest) with ID details. Some people find that this method of identification suits their needs.

Helpful hints

- If you have to fill in any medical details on the ID, ask your GP or allergy specialist to help you, or to check what you have written.
- ID should be carried at all times.
- ID should be visible.
- The information provided on the ID should be correct and up to date.
- If you are travelling to a foreign country, the ID should be modified or alternative information provided so that the people there can understand it (see Chapter 16, 'Holidays and Travelling').
- If your ID carries a yearly fee, make sure that this is paid (perhaps by Direct Debit), so that your details remain on the database. Failure to pay could render your ID invalid.

Although these seem very obvious points, they are often overlooked!

6
Food Allergy and Going to School

Anaphylaxis is relatively rare, whereas food allergy causing very unpleasant but not life-threatening symptoms is common. Bear in mind, too, that the severity of allergic reactions can change over time. This chapter deals with the serious, possibly life-threatening, allergic reaction that might affect your child when at school.

PRE-SCHOOL

Pre-school children are usually too young to know how to avoid foods to which they are allergic. Food is usually a large part of their day, which is broken up by snack and meal breaks. As the child's parents, you play a key role in managing this. It is your responsibility to make sure that there are suitable snacks and treats available for everyday activities and special activities. You should liaise closely with the class teacher and the parents of the other children. As always, it is essential to have an action plan for emergency use, which should be reviewed regularly.

Some nurseries and pre-schools ask for a letter from your child's doctor, confirming the allergy.

MEDICAL QUESTIONNAIRE

Parents are usually required to complete a medical questionnaire when their child joins a new school. It will include questions that are designed to identify children with allergies to foods.

A child at risk of anaphylaxis presents a challenge to any school. However, with the correct plans, information and co-ordination, school life can continue as normal. Each child should have an action plan devised for use in an emergency.

SETTING UP AN ACTION PLAN

For a child who has a severe food allergy, the parents, teachers and others will make considerable efforts to try to ensure that as many risks as possible are reduced. A good website is www.allergyinschools.org.uk which has very useful and detailed information. However, with the best will in the world, accidents can still happen. If they do, it is essential that everyone around at the time knows what to expect and what is expected of them.

Child-specific action plan

Sample child-specific action plans (or protocols) are available from the Anaphylaxis Campaign and from the allergyinschools website mentioned above. They have a standard format and will help you to complete a plan that is specific to your child. The best way to achieve this is to formulate a plan in association with the school nurse, the nursery/school staff, the head teacher, the allergy specialist, the GP, the school health and safety co-ordinator and the local education authority. The final version should then be distributed to everyone concerned.

The plan deals with all of the important issues, including:

- Anaphylaxis – what it is, and why a protocol is required to ensure the child's safety.
- Identification – ensuring that the child is known to be at risk.
- Consent and agreement – between the parents or guardians and the school.
- Emergency procedure – the action to take, including guidance on administering adrenaline and obtaining medical help (dialling 999).
- Food management – how to prevent reactions.
- Medication – antihistamines, adrenaline.
- Professional indemnity – for school staff willing to give emergency treatment.
- Reducing the risks – the emergency/action plan, having role-play periodically (e.g. every term).
- Staff training – relevant literature and videos/DVDs about the allergy, having role-play, training in administering the medication.
- What to tell the other children.

The plan is in place not only for your child's safety but also to help the school staff, and will bring with it security and assurance. It is helpful if the plan is role-played periodically so as to aid speed and understanding in the event of an anaphylactic reaction.

Action For Anaphylaxis is a video available from the Anaphylaxis Campaign. It is about a child having an anaphylactic reaction at school and how it was managed successfully – using an action plan. It would be useful for the school to obtain a copy of this for training purposes. Bring it to the attention of the school staff when you are formulating the action plan, as they may be unaware of its existence. Tell them also about the information that is available from the Anaphylaxis Campaign, which they might find useful, and about the Campaign's website (all contact details in Appendix 1).

Copies of the action plan should be held by the school, the parents, the GP and the local education authority. It is essential that all parties be kept informed of any changes and agree any amendments. The action plan should have the date clearly marked so that old versions can be discarded and do not get mixed up with the updates.

Government Guidance

Managing Medicines in Schools and Early Years Settings is a document published by the Department for Education and Skills and the Department of Health. It includes contributions from patient-support groups such as the Anaphylaxis Campaign, and sets out a framework within which local authorities, local health trusts, schools and early-years organisations can work together to develop policies to ensure that children requiring medicines receive appropriate support. It can be obtained, free, from the Department for Education and Skills (see Appendix 1).

Wales, Scotland and Northern Ireland have similar guidance.

HEALTH AND SAFETY IN SCHOOL

It is the duty of school staff to safeguard the health of pupils. Although teachers have a general legal duty to act on behalf of the parents (*in loco parentis*) they are *not* responsible for administering or supervising pupils taking medication. Some staff may, however, volunteer to undertake appropriate training to enable them to do so.

All schools are required to have a policy for calling an ambulance if it is required. Treatment will usually begin when the ambulance staff

Summary of action to take for a severe reaction

Action	Reason
Delegate someone to call 999 for an ambulance, stating that the child is having an anaphylactic reaction	So you may stay with and reassure the child
Lie the child down on his or her back, immediately	To minimise the drop in blood pressure that is characteristic of an anaphylactic reaction and to increase blood flow to the brain
Give adrenaline if there is: difficulty in breathing or speaking or swallowing; or a feeling of faintness or weakness; or collapse	To reverse the symptoms of anaphylaxis
Delegate someone to call the parents (do not leave the child alone)	To keep parents informed and so they come to provide support for the child as soon as possible
On arrival of the ambulance: parent (or staff member if the parent is not there) to go in the ambulance to nearest A&E department	Support for the child and to provide information to medical staff about the child and the reaction/treatment given

arrive; this is appropriate for most incidents. There are, however, certain conditions that require immediate treatment and cannot wait for the ambulance. One such condition is anaphylaxis.

Medical training of school staff

This is usually done by the GP, school doctor, school nurse or paediatrician, and sometimes by the community paediatric nurse or health visitor. Teachers will have the opportunity to practise giving the injections and to have their questions answered. The agreed action plan may also be discussed. Certificates of competence are sometimes given. There are no formal nationally agreed standards, so training will vary.

If this training has not been carried out in your child's school, ask your GP to contact the school nurse, who will arrange for it to be done.

Issues for the school staff

Indemnity for school staff is an important issue, and the lack of it has, in the past, discouraged many from volunteering to administer medication. The teachers' unions advise their members that, if they agree to take on this responsibility, they should follow strictly controlled guidelines and obtain professional indemnity from their employers, to cover them in cases of alleged negligence.

The school or the local education authority often provides indemnity as a matter of course. It is the responsibility of individual school staff members to ensure they are fully covered for action they might take within the scope of their employment.

Medication at school

Schools have their own policy on the storage of medication. They may allow pupils to carry it if they are of an appropriate age, or it may be held by the class teacher or in the secretaries' office. On no account should it be kept in a locked cupboard, because there might be a delay in getting it if the keys cannot be located. It would be wise for you to check the school's policy and, if necessary, negotiate a suitable compromise.

Some schools have a policy of locking away all medication. The main reasons for this are worries that the child will lose the medication or that it will be misused by another child. If your child's school has such a policy, discuss it with the head teacher. It may also be worth getting the GP to write to the head teacher with his or her recommendations regarding your child carrying the medication or where and how medication should be stored at school.

RECORDS

It is essential that a record be kept of any allergic reaction that occurs. The information should be dated and signed by the staff involved in the treatment. Details of mild and more severe reactions and their causes, location, etc., can be useful in preventing future reactions. For example, if every reaction happens at lunch time despite your child taking a packed lunch from home, it could indicate that sandwiches are being swapped.

FOOD AT SCHOOL

It is understandable that you may be concerned about your child eating in a place where there can be potentially harmful foods around. However, eating with friends is an important part of fitting in and social integration.

Although some parents prefer to supply all their child's food for consumption at school, others are happy to trust the school caterers to provide suitable food. It is sensible, though, to formulate a code of practice that will encompass a particular child's special dietary needs and ensure that only correct food is provided. The Anaphylaxis Campaign can help with this.

To handle the growing problem of pupils with food allergy, some schools create a peanut/nut-free or milk-free table for children to eat at. They also establish a no-food-trading policy, as children swapping food with each other is a major reason for allergic reactions at school.

Make sure that your child knows what foods cause an allergic reaction and the importance of avoiding them. Role-play possible scenarios to help your child feel confident when dealing with situations relating to eating and the allergy – for example, peer pressure, teasing, bullying or just the temptation to eat an offending food.

Sometimes the will to protect children physically can result in harming them psychologically. So it is difficult – but important – to get the balance right. There are many ways of keeping others informed about your child's allergy, including:

- educating your child not to accept food from others,
- joining an allergy support group,
- talking to people, explaining about the allergy,
- using the Anaphylaxis Campaign literature, videos/DVDs and websites.

Before your child attends a new school, schedule a meeting with the teachers, school nurse, catering staff and office staff. Explain to them about the allergy, which foods cause a reaction and precautions that must be taken. They should also be told about the emergency procedure (the action plan) that should be followed, reading food labels and lunch time considerations such as:

- who sits with whom, and with which food,
- going home for lunch,

- your attending at lunch time to supervise,
- whether your child should eat food provided by the school or bring food from home.

Banning foods from the school: the disadvantages

Banning a particular food is one option in a school's management of food allergies. Doing this can, however, have associated problems:

- It creates a false sense of security, because pupils feel confident to eat any foods that are offered to them at school, when staff do not realise that it is not just peanut butter and Snickers that contain nut/peanut derivatives.
- Some parents might see this as an imposition, especially if it is going to be disadvantageous to their child. For example, nuts/peanuts are an important source of protein for vegetarians or vegans, or an underweight fussy child will eat only peanut butter sandwiches. Bans are likely to leave parents feeling cross rather than creating a harmonious, safe environment for the allergic child.
- For a ban to work effectively, everyone involved would have to constantly read food labels. This might be unrealistic and therefore unachievable.
- If all parents of children with severe food allergies requested that the offending foods be removed from the school, the resulting diet would become very limited and everyone would be confused as well as irate!
- Creating a ban might stigmatise the allergic child.
- Banning a food from the school creates a false situation and does not teach the child how to live with the allergy. When they eventually leave school they will be unprepared for life in the real world.

SCHOOL ACTIVITIES

Review plans for any activities that may involve food (e.g. parties, trips, cooking, crafts) on a monthly or half-term basis so that plans can be made to allow your child to participate in them safely. If your child is to go on a school trip, make sure that everyone involved in providing refreshments on the outing is given plenty of notice about suitable food and drink.

Unsuitable activities

Certain class activities – for example, cookery classes, craft lessons, custard pie competition (!) – may be unsafe. It is important that children who cannot take part in these activities are given related alternative tasks. Otherwise, both they and their fellow pupils might feel alienated. Work with the school staff to find a suitable solution to this sort of problem.

7
Food Allergy
in Young Adults

It is a fact that anaphylaxis resulting from food allergy can be fatal, although this is very rare. In recent years the victims have tended to be young people in their late teens or early twenties. Perhaps this is partly because people in this age group tend to take more risks or are more susceptible to peer pressure to 'fit in'. Whatever the reason, it has become tragically apparent that some lives could have been saved if the victims had had a greater understanding of their condition, had carried adrenaline with them and had taken more care in selecting food when eating away from home.

Recognising these facts, the Anaphylaxis Campaign has distributed thousands of information booklets to students throughout the UK. The booklet gives the following tips to help people with a severe allergy to live a normal and full life:

- Face up to your allergy – don't ignore it, hoping it will go away.
- Read food labels. It takes only seconds and could save your life.
- When eating out, be direct with waiters and catering staff.
- Avoid eating in high-risk places: for example, the food in Indian and Oriental restaurants often has nuts and peanuts among the ingredients, and misunderstandings can occur among staff who don't speak much English.
- Don't handle this alone – educate your friends about your allergy.
- Be alert to all symptoms. Don't ignore them.
- If you have an adrenaline kit, make sure you take it everywhere.

The Anaphylaxis Campaign runs workshops and education groups designed to help young people who are at risk of anaphylaxis to understand and manage their allergy and to develop confidence. The information should help them in the everyday situations that can put them at risk as well as showing how to avoid needless restrictions.

This knowledge should reduce the incidence of both anaphylaxis and fatalities: if a reaction does occur, the adrenaline will be readily available and administered correctly.

COLLEGE STUDENTS LIVING-IN

If you are a college or university student, you should inform staff, room mates and hall mates about the foods that cause an allergic reaction, symptoms to be aware of and action to take if a reaction occurs.

Keep your medication in an easily accessible place, and a laminated up-to-date action plan by the phone.

EXTRA TIPS

- Too much alcohol can affect your judgement and speed up an allergic reaction, so beware!
- Before you kiss, check what your partner has been eating; it may be unsafe to do so until they have washed and cleaned their teeth.
- Exercise can speed up the rate of a reaction; slow down if you suspect a reaction may be coming on.
- A food to which you are allergic can turn up unexpectedly, so always check food ingredient labels. If there is no label, don't eat the food but find something that is definitely safe for you to eat.
- Put yourself in your friends' position. Would you find it a problem if they told you they have to be careful about what they eat and have to carry medication around just in case they eat something they shouldn't? And, by the way, could you learn how to administer it just in case they are too ill? Would you mind? Of course not! In fact, you would probably feel quite pleased that you were trusted to do this important task.

If you want more information, try the various websites listed in Appendix 2; for example, www.allergyaction.org has lots of ideas. Some websites have pages dedicated to teenagers and young adults.

Enjoying Food

8
The Dietitian's Role

If you wish to see a dietitian for dietary advice, you need a referral from either your GP or a hospital consultant. Any hospital consultant or GP can refer a patient to the dietitian but it is usually done by a dermatologist, chest physician or allergy specialist because they are the specialists who see the people with allergies.

Every child on a restricted diet should be referred to a paediatric dietitian for assessment and advice.

GETTING A REFERRAL

Even if you decide to see a dietitian privately, you still need a doctor's referral. This is to protect you from dietary advice that might adversely affect an ongoing medical condition or treatment. After your appointment, it is usual for the dietitian to send a letter to the referring doctor to inform them of the nutritional advice you have been given. The doctor then files this information in your medical notes for future reference.

Unfortunately, some people choose to see a 'nutritionist', 'nutritional therapist' or similar person who may have only very limited or no medical qualifications. In addition, they are not registered with the Health Professionals Council (HPC) and are therefore not bound by any national regulations. You do not need a doctor's referral to see them, and their treatment may be damaging if they do not know your full medical history. The other drawback is that follow-up care may not be given after you are placed on a restricted diet, which is dangerous. The following scenario is more common than is often realised.

Julie has had allergy testing by an 'alternative' therapist and has been told to avoid all dairy products, wheat, red meat, citrus fruits and soya. Without follow-up care by a medically qualified person, she has remained on a restricted diet for some time, believing that it is good for her health. It is only when Julie begins to feel unwell and goes to her GP for advice that she is referred to a dietitian for 'unexplained weight loss and anaemia' and she is diagnosed with malnutrition.

Such potentially harmful consequences can occur because:

- the poorly qualified/unqualified 'therapist' has a poor knowledge and understanding of the possible nutritional implications of placing someone on a restricted diet and not giving them follow-up care for prolonged periods of time,
- the individual has a poor understanding of the prescribed diet and may not realise that new symptoms are related to it,
- the individual cannot afford to go back and see the 'therapist' for on-going care.

This is why it is essential to see a fully qualified dietitian.

Remember that anyone – adult or child – cutting major food groups out of their diet is at risk of malnutrition and needs advice from a qualified professional.

SEEING THE DIETITIAN

When you go to see the dietitian, it will be useful if you are prepared and know what to expect so that you can get the most from your visit.

Obvious food allergy

If you have had a severe allergic reaction to food and the allergen causing it was easily identifiable, the dietitian will advise you about completely excluding that food and its derivatives from your diet, and will suggest replacement foods to maintain good health.

Hidden food allergy

If you have had a severe allergic reaction but the cause was unknown, you will have been referred for allergy testing (see Chapters 2 and 3) before you see the dietitian. Once the likely cause of the allergy has been identified, the dietitian will advise you on how to avoid the culprit and its derivatives whilst maintaining a balanced diet.

Factors to discuss with your dietitian

When you are going to embark on a special diet, discuss with your dietitian:

- the aim of the diet, to make sure you understand it and how to follow it,
- the likely cost of the foods (they can be considerably more expensive than 'ordinary' food),
- how to make sure that your diet is nutritious,
- how long you will be on the diet,
- how to manage when eating out, including holidays, business travel, work lunches, celebrations and social events,
- what treats you are allowed,
- your general health,
- any medication that you are taking (e.g. antihistamines) and whether you carry adrenaline with you at all times,
- how often you should contact the dietitian,
- how much support the dietitian will be able to give you and when.

The dietitian will be able to advise you or give you information about many aspects. The list below is in alphabetical order, and the importance of the entries will be specific to your particular needs.

- adapting existing recipes,
- baby formulas,
- comprehensive list of foods to avoid,
- contact by phone in case of queries,
- cookbooks, new recipes and cooking tips,
- eating away from home/celebrations,
- encouragement and support,
- food manufacturers' information and 'free from' lists,
- ideas to help add variety and palatability to your diet,
- information on food labelling to aid understanding and interpretation,
- nutrient supplementation,
- nutritional adequacy of your diet, diet sheets and meal plans,
- products available on prescription,
- replacement or substitute foods and where to buy them,
- review appointments,
- supermarket 'free from' lists,
- support groups,
- translations of food information, for travelling abroad,
- written advice as required.

Factors that you need to consider when following a restricted diet include:

- being organised about food shopping and cooking,
- shopping: location and opening hours of specialist shops, and which substitute foods to buy,
- having confidence to explain your needs,
- your cooking skills – to adapt recipes,
- the cost of your diet,
- your feelings of deprivation,
- social isolation,
- whether meals should be kept separate or all the family to eat the same food,
- nutrition,
- taste: acceptability of substitute foods.

In recent years, many 'special diet' foods have become more available, accessible and acceptable. There has been a general improvement in both their taste and their price.

9
Food Labelling

If you are allergic to a food, it is relatively easy to avoid it in its natural state. Avoiding derivatives of that food, however, is more difficult. This chapter discusses current food-labelling laws and initiatives by the food industry that will help you to identify and choose suitable foods for your special diet.

Since the improved food labelling regulations were implemented in November 2005, it has been much easier to identify foods sold within the EU that contain any of the 12 major food allergens. The regulations state that the presence of the allergen must be clear to the consumer. Foods sold outside the EU are not bound by the same regulations, and allergens may be hidden or omitted from the ingredients label, assuming that the product has one at all.

Products manufactured and labelled after 25 November 2004 (manufacturers were given a year in which to make their labelling comply with the regulations) must be in line with the new legislation. Products manufactured and labelled before that date may continue to be sold while stocks last.

PRODUCT CHANGES

Manufacturers sometimes alter the formulation of their products. This may happen when a supplier changes or with recipe developments. This change can result in a previously safe food becoming unsafe. Because of this, it is essential that you check labels *every* time, even if you have had the product before.

It is also worth noting that the ingredients may differ, depending on the country in which a product is manufactured. So if you are in France and see a product you usually eat in the UK, don't assume that it will be suitable.

FOOD ALLERGEN LABELLING LAWS

Since November 2005 pre-packaged foods sold within the EU are required by law to indicate the presence of 12 major allergens if they are deliberately included in the product. These 12 allergens are:

- cow's milk
- eggs
- fish
- crustaceans
- sesame
- gluten-containing cereals (wheat, rye, barley, oats, spelt, kamut and their hybridised strains)
- peanuts
- nuts (almond, hazelnut, cashew, pecan, Brazil, pistachio, macadamia, Queensland nut)
- soyabean
- mustard
- celery
- sulphur dioxide and sulphites (more than 10mg/kg or 10mg/litre), expressed as SO_2

At the end of 2007, lupin and molluscs will be added to the list, making a total of 14.

Allergens not on this list will have to be labelled in most cases but there are exceptions. For more information get in touch with the Food Standards Agency (contact details in Appendix 1).

The legislation applies only to packaged manufactured foods sold in the EU. Exemptions to these laws include foods sold loose, such as bakery or butchery products and delicatessen goods. (These are also at risk of cross-contamination: see Chapter 15.)

ALCOHOLIC DRINKS

Only drinks with more than 1.2% alcohol content are required to be labelled if they contain any of the 12 allergens listed above. Other ingredients remain legally undeclared.

'MAY CONTAIN' ISSUES

The labelling covers only ingredients added intentionally and not traces that may be present due to cross-contamination. An increasing number of food manufacturers are adding to their packaging the declaration 'This product may contain traces of nuts/peanuts' or

'Made on a production line/in a factory handling nuts/peanuts' (or other allergenic ingredients). The aim is to highlight products that might have been in contact with that allergen – for example, by being baked in a contaminated tin or by passing along a contaminated production line (see also Chapter 15, 'Cross-contamination').

In some instances, such a label may be put on a product even if the chance of cross-contamination is minuscule. This has resulted in many products that do not contain nuts/peanuts, and were previously suitable for someone allergic to nuts/peanuts, now becoming out of bounds. The public's response to this practice has not been favourable, because it has reduced the food choices available to anyone with that food allergy. Some people are therefore now unnecessarily avoiding foods that were previously regarded as – and may still be – safe.

On the other hand, many people choose to ignore 'may contain' labels, believing they are a cop-out and don't represent a real risk. This labelling puts the onus on the consumer to assess the risk and make a decision as to whether they will eat the product based on the limited amount of information given. This is not sensible and you should always heed such labels. In practice, there have been incidents where ignoring the 'may contain' label has led to severe reactions.

In 2006 the Food Standards Agency (see below) produced a guidance document on best practice for the food industry regarding these and other manufacturing issues concerned with food allergies. A summary document of this guidance is to be produced for smaller food-manufacturing businesses.

The food industry's response to the food allergy issues

Several widely publicised fatalities linked to food allergies (nut/peanut allergies in particular), and the formation of the Anaphylaxis Campaign in 1994, have led to an increased awareness among the food industry, the public and health professionals about food allergy issues and implications.

The food industry as a whole has made some positive progress in addressing some of the issues. These include:

- improved food ingredient labelling of products,
- availability of 'free from' lists,
- voluntary allergen advice panel on food labels,
- new production and distribution practices at manufacture and retailer level,

- increased range of special diet foods available,
- compliance with food labelling legislation,
- more specific information on food labels about the risks of cross-contamination of food allergens during production, including the use of 'may contain' labelling.

THE FOOD AND DRINK FEDERATION

The Food and Drink Federation (FDF) represents the UK food and drink manufacturing industry. The members work in partnership to help ensure that our food is safe in all aspects, including identification and control of major food allergens. Members of the Federation are food and drink manufacturing companies and trade associations dealing with specific food and drink sectors.

THE FOOD STANDARDS AGENCY

The Food Standards Agency (FSA) is a government-funded agency that was set up in 2000 by an Act of Parliament to protect the public's health and consumer interests in relation to food.

The FSA has a dedicated food allergy and intolerance team. The team's website has useful information on many types of food allergies and intolerances, as well as information for consumers on eating out, buying food and current food labelling legislation. Specific consumer queries about nutrition can be answered by the team, by phone, email or letter (contact details in Appendix 1). They do not give advice on diagnosis and diet plans; this information should be sought from dietitians or other health professionals.

In 2006 the FSA produced an advice and information document for food manufacturers: *Guidance on Allergen Management and Consumer Information: best practice guidance on managing food allergens with particular reference to avoiding cross-contamination and using appropriate advisory labelling.* It can be ordered from the FSA or downloaded from its website.

TRADING STANDARDS

Trading Standards officers and Environmental Health officers are responsible for enforcing food-labelling laws. They should be contacted if a food is labelled incorrectly – for example, if you have an allergic reaction to a food that, according to the ingredients label, is safe for you. The Trading Standards officer will obtain a sample of the product and analyse it in the laboratory to check for an undeclared ingredient on the label – based on your evidence.

SUPERMARKET FOOD-ALLERGEN LABELLING

Many supermarkets now have a labelling policy that is designed to help people with an allergy to read food labels. Customers are able to see at a glance whether products are suitable for a particular diet; for example, cow's-milk-free, nut-free, egg-free and wheat-free. The information is often in a panel or box, as part of the food labelling. It sometimes contains an easy-to-spot graphic such as an ear of corn to indicate that the product is suitable for a gluten-free diet, or a cow with a cross through it to indicate that the product is suitable for a cow's-milk-free diet. A possible drawback is that consumers might then not read the ingredients panel.

Some food shops also have a panel on the packaging saying that the product contains, for example, wheat or nuts.

'Free from' lists

Most major supermarkets and many food manufacturers now voluntarily hold detailed lists of own-brand products that are free from all the major allergens, such as milk, nuts or eggs. They will even sometimes compile a tailor-made list if you have more than one allergy. The supermarket head office or in-store customer services section will be able to advise you about this.

The 'free from' lists are an excellent guide, but, because errors or changes may occur, you must always read the food labels and ingredients listings as well to be sure that the foods are indeed safe for you.

FOOD OUTLETS

At present there is no legal requirement for any catering outlet to give information about what has gone into the food on sale. However, many fast-food outlets now produce information on food ingredients. For example, McDonald's produces and has readily available a full ingredients listing for every product it sells.

Some fast-food outlets also keep food items separate from one another. This considerably reduces the risk of cross-contamination (see Chapter 15) and, if you decide to eat out, it would be safer for you to eat in places that follow this practice. For more information about eating out, see Chapter 14 ('Eating Away from Home').

COSMETICS LABELLING

The sixth amendment to the European Union Cosmetic Directive (1993) was implemented in December 1997. It requires the ingredi-

Table 9.1 Ingredients and their INCI names (as used on product packaging)

Ingredient	INCI name
Avocado	*Persea gratissima*
Bitter almond	*Prunus amara*
Brazil nut	*Bertholletia excelsa*
Coconut	*Cocos nucifera*
Cod liver oil	*Gadi iecur*
Egg	*Ovum*
Hazel nut	*Corylus rostrata/americana/avellana*
Macadamia nut	*Macademia ternifolia*
Melon	*Cucumis melo*
Milk	*Lac*
Mixed fish oil	*Piscum iecur*
Pea	*Pisum sativum*
Peanut oil	Arachis oil [*Arachis hypogaea*]
Sesame	*Sesamum indicum*
Soya	*Glycine soja*
Sweet almond/Almond oil	*Prunus dulcis*
Walnut	*Juglans regia/nigra*
Whey protein	*Lactis proteinum*

ents to be included in the label for soaps, cosmetics and 'personal care products'. This classification is taken to include any preparation that is applied to the skin, eyes, mouth, hair or nails for the purpose of cleansing, giving a pleasant smell or enhancing appearance. The labelling has helped consumers to identify products that might be harmful to them. However, because the labelling is in Latin, it is sometimes incomprehensible to the layperson. This can cause a problem when common ingredients are not recognised. An example of this is 'arachis oil', which is the International Nomenclature of Cosmetic Ingredients (INCI) name for peanut oil.

The only answer is for you to have a list with the Latin names of the ingredients that you must avoid and refer to this whenever buying products. Remember that allergens may be present in sample and tester products in-store. Note, too, that nut and seed oils are used in spray format and can be inhaled straight into the lungs, whilst many shampoos and conditioners contain recognised food allergens, including nuts, seeds, wheat, milk, egg and a wide range of fruits.

The Cosmetic Toiletry and Perfumery Association Ltd is prepared to answer queries about these issues and has a useful leaflet listing some of the Latin (INCI) names. Table 9.1 is a list of some of the ordinary names and their Latin names.

A comprehensive inventory of these substances is available from the Cosmetic Toiletry and Perfumery Association website (see Appendix 2).

Within the EU the terminology used in the labelling of these products must comply with that in the inventory.

10
Special Diets

The major sections in this chapter have information and advice about specific special diets. The foods included are those that most commonly cause allergic reactions in the European Union. This is a reflection of the 2005 legislation that amended the rules about the inclusion of food allergens in ingredient labels.

Advice is given in this chapter on how to ensure adequate nutrition while following these avoidance diets successfully.

Some people think they are already following a special diet and totally avoiding a food when they are unknowingly consuming hidden components of that food. This may be due to:

- poor understanding of food labels,
- not reading food labels,
- eating foods abroad where food labels do not list all ingredients,
- eating foods that do not carry a label, such as bakery, delicatessen and butchery products,
- eating foods prepared by someone who is unaware of or does not understand the person's needs,
- cross-contamination.

Unwittingly eating 'hidden' ingredients may account for a reaction of 'unknown origin'. Once this is clarified, a clear diagnosis usually becomes apparent.

Following an avoidance diet may not be as difficult as you might first think. There may even be some positive changes to your diet, such as new recipe ideas and the chance to experiment with some new foods. Also remember that a lot of the foods and dishes you ate before your diagnosis will still be suitable, or at least will require only a slight adaptation.

Even if you hate cooking, there are lots of foods you can still enjoy – this chapter will give you some ideas. The major change will be the fact that you have to take responsibility for your own diet from now on. You can no longer just accept food that is offered to you without discussing your requirements with the host – including issues of cross-contamination that may well have been overlooked. Sometimes it may just be easier, safer or more appropriate to take your own food or eat before you go out.

For specific dietary advice you should always seek a referral to see a dietitian. This is especially important for children, who have high nutritional requirements for growth and development. (See Chapter 8.)

COW'S-MILK- AND DAIRY-FREE DIET

There is a lot of confusion and misinformation about foods considered to be 'dairy'. Essentially dairy food is cow's milk and its derivatives such as cheese, cream, yoghurt and fromage frais.

Many processed foods contain dairy products. These are easily identified in dairy-based foods such as cheesecake or rice pudding; it is the 'hidden' milk is in products that are more difficult to recognise.

Since November 2005, however, milk and milk derivatives have had to be clearly labelled on all pre-packed foods sold within the European Union (see Chapter 9, 'Food Labelling'). It is therefore important to avoid foods sold loose, such as bakery or butchery products and delicatessen items, where the ingredients are not listed and could therefore contain milk or its derivatives. Foods sold outside the EU do not necessarily have the same labelling laws, so extreme caution is essential before consuming these. Milk derivatives you need to check labels for include:

- butter, butter oil, buttermilk,
- casein, caseinates, hydrolysed casein, sodium caseinate,
- cheese, cream cheese,
- cow's milk (fresh, UHT, evaporated, condensed, dried),
- cream, sour cream,
- curd,
- flavourings.*
- ghee,
- lactoglobulin,

---

* Foods sold outside the EU may include 'flavourings' on the product ingredients list. This may be a milk-derived flavouring such as sodium caseinate or lactose which is used as a flavour carrier. It is recommended that you avoid flavourings if you have a severe allergy to milk. (Within the EU, milk-derived flavouring will state this on the label.)

- lactose,
- milk solids,
- quark,
- whey, hydrolysed whey, whey powder, whey syrup sweetener,
- yoghurt, fromage frais,

Approximately 2–4% of young children have an allergy to dairy products. The good news is that around 95% of them will have outgrown the allergy by the age of 5 years.

What about milk from other animals?
The allergenic proteins in milk from mammals such as goat, sheep, buffalo and horse are very similar to those in cow's milk and can therefore cause similar reactions. So they should all be avoided on a cow's-milk-free diet unless you are already tolerating them or unless advised otherwise by your allergy specialist.

Replacement foods and ingredients
As with any special diet, you can make it more appealing, varied and nutritious by using replacement ingredients and specially formulated products. Table 10.1 gives you examples.

Recipes for home-made non-dairy products can be found in any vegan or dairy-free cookbook (see Appendix 3).

Table 10.1 Replacements for milk products

Instead of	Choose
Cow's milk	Soya, rice, oat, nut, pea, chufa, potato or quinoa milks
Butter	Soya or milk-free spread
Dairy hard cheese	Soya cheese
Dairy cream cheese	Soya cream cheese
Dairy ice-cream	Soya or oat ice-cream
Dairy yoghurt	Soya yoghurt
Cream	Soya or oat cream, coconut milk*

* Check the ingredients because, occasionally, coconut milks contain cow's milk derivatives.

The end of this section gives lists of replacement products that are available. It really is worth trying them and including them in your diet – you will be surprised by how good they are. Experiment with them in new recipes or adapt existing recipes.

The products listed were correct at the time of writing but remember *always* to read their food labels before you eat them. Remember, too, that new products are always becoming available, so if you just use my lists you may be missing out!

DAIRY-FREE DIET AND NUTRITION

Table 10.2 outlines the recommended daily calcium requirements for children and adults. By using the replacement foods listed in Table 10.3 you will be able to achieve adequate nutrition from your dairy-free diet. However, a dairy-free diet without these replacement foods is likely to be nutritionally deficient. It is always advisable to seek advice from a dietitian before you remove foods from your diet, especially staple foods such as milk. (Chapter 8 discusses how to get a referral to a dietitian.)

Table 10.2 Daily calcium requirements

Age group	Calcium requirements
0–1 year	525mg
1–3 years	350mg
4–6 years	450mg
7–10 years	550mg
Males 11–18 years	1,000mg
Males 19+ years	700mg
Females 11–18 years	800mg
Females 19+ years	700mg

A woman who is breast-feeding requires an extra 550mg

Calcium

Dairy foods are usually the main source of calcium in your diet, which is essential for the development of strong bones and teeth, normal blood clotting, nerve function and enzyme activity. It is especially important in children and adolescents but is in fact an essential nutrient throughout life. Women who are breast-feeding have a very high requirement. It is thought that adequate calcium in early life may help protect against osteoporosis ('brittle' bones) later on.

Calcium supplements

For days that you are not able to achieve your requirements, speak to your dietitian about the most suitable calcium supplement. Syrup, effervescent and chewable calcium supplements are most suitable for children. Adults may prefer to take it in tablet form.

For optimum absorption of the calcium in your diet, vitamin D is required. This is made naturally in your skin when it is exposed to sunlight. Any calcium supplement should therefore contain vitamin D as well unless there is a good supply in the diet.

Dietary sources of vitamin D include oily fish (sardines, mackerel), eggs, offal and vitamin D-enriched foods such as margarine and breakfast cereals.

If you are on a restricted diet, particularly a milk-free diet, it is recommended that you make use of alternative foods such as calcium-enriched soya milks, cheeses and yoghurts, and try to eat foods rich in calcium to ensure an adequate intake. Note that organic products are *not* calcium-enriched.

Kosher foods

Orthodox Jews do not consume milk and meat together, so many foods they eat are specifically prepared to be milk-free. Many of these foods, particularly the 'supervised' kosher foods, are suitable for people with a severe milk allergy. Similarly, many of the 'meat' restaurants do not have any dairy or dairy derivatives on the premises, providing a safe environment for someone with a severe milk allergy.

The Really Jewish Food Guide gives detailed information about these issues. For details of this and all other matters concerning the kosher diet and philosophy, contact London Beth Din(details in Appendix 1).

Table 10.3 Calcium content of foods (average portions)

Dairy and non-dairy foods

1 glass/200ml cow's milk	240mg
1 glass/200ml soya milk (not enriched)	25mg
1 glass/200ml calcium-enriched soya milk*	250mg
1 glass/200ml rice milk*	26mg
1 glass/200ml calcium-enriched rice milk	240mg
1 glass/200ml oat milk*	0mg
1 glass/200ml calcium-enriched oat milk	240mg
1 glass/200ml pea milk*	84mg
1 glass/200ml almond milk*	32mg
1 glass/200ml Lactolite (low lactose milk)	240mg
30g dairy hard cheese	220mg
30g soya hard cheese *	25mg
30g dairy cream cheese	30mg
30g soya cream cheese*	25mg
125mg dairy yoghurt	200mg
125g soya yoghurt*	125mg
50g/small pot fromage frais	44mg
1 glass/200ml calcium fortified orange juice	245mg
1 glass/200ml calcium-fortified water	60mg
1 glass/200ml tap water (not boiled or filtered)	22mg

*The amount of calcium in these products may vary – check the product label.

Table 10.3 Calcium content of foods (average portions) *continued*

Other foods

100g sardines (tinned, bones are eaten)	500mg
30g fortified porridge (before milk added)	400mg
50g tofu (soya bean curd)	255mg
100g/1 large bowl muesli	200mg
3 dried figs	170mg
100g spinach	160mg
2 heaped tablespoon red kidney beans	100mg
100g/3 slices white bread	100mg
30g breakfast cereals	100mg
25g/7 whole Brazil nuts	90mg
60g shelled prawns	90mg
14g/1 tablespoon sunflower/sesame seeds	85mg
1 medium orange	75mg
150g/1 very small tin baked beans	75mg
25g/12 whole almonds	65mg
25g/¼ bunch watercress	55mg
100g/3 slices wholemeal bread	50mg
100g green vegetables	50mg

*The amount of calcium in these products may vary – check the product label.

Note that dairy-replacement products that are not calcium-enriched contain little or no calcium, so aim to choose ones that are calcium-enriched.

Sex

It may be useful to know that most condoms contain casein, a milk protein. If you are very sensitive to traces of milk, this could be an issue for you to consider. Details of casein-free condoms are available from the Vegan Society (contact details in Appendix 1).

Medication

Lots of medications contain lactose and other milk derivatives. Always check the ingredients or ask your pharmacist to do so.

Never assume that, because your doctor has prescribed your medication, it will be milk-free. It has been known for doctors to prescribe antihistamines containing milk derivatives for someone with a severe milk allergy to use in an allergic reaction to milk! To be safe:

- Check the ingredients of all prescribed and over-the-counter medications before taking them.
- Remember that medicines are often reformulated, so you need to check ingredients every time you open a new packet.
- Do not take a medication that has no ingredients label with it until you have checked the ingredients with your pharmacist. If you are unable to do this, do not take it.
- If you are admitted to hospital, do not assume that the staff will always remember to check that all prescribed medication is milk-free. Make sure you remind them of your requirements.

Toiletries and cosmetics

Toiletries and cosmetics often contain cow's milk derivatives. See Chapter 9 ('Food Labelling') to find out how you can identify these products.

Sweeteners

Sweeteners often contain lactose. Remember to check the ingredients of the sweeteners offered to you, whether in granulated or in tablet form.

'Whiteners' in tea and coffee

Tea and coffee 'whiteners' are usually cow's-milk based.

Soya milk tends to separate or curdle when added to tea or coffee. Cooling the drink a little first sometimes reduces this. Look in a vegan cookbook for information on how you can prevent this, or alternatively do some experiments of your own.

Glucono delta lactone

This is a form of sugar found in grapes, and is commonly used in breadmaking when yeast has to be avoided. Although the name is deceptive, it *does not* contain lactose or cow's milk.

REPLACEMENT FOODS

The information that follows is only a guide. The products listed can be found in a variety of places – although availability will depend on the vendor. Healthfood shops, supermarkets and distribution companies such as Goodness Direct and Dietary Needs Direct (contact details in Appendix 1) are excellent places to shop for your special diet products.

Remember that you should always read the ingredients labels thoroughly. If you are in doubt as to whether a product is suitable, please contact the manufacturer.

Soya milks

Allergycare	Soya shake powder: banana, vanilla, strawberry, coconut
Alpro Soya	Fresh and longlife; sweetened and unsweetened; regular and light; flavoured mini milks: chocolate, vanilla, strawberry; with added calcium and vitamins; organic (no added calcium)
Evernat	Organic soya milk
Granose & Whitewave (Haldane Foods)	In a variety of sizes: calcium-enriched; organic; sweetened and unsweetened
Granovita	Added calcium, organic, sugar-free
Plamil	Sweetened; unsweetened; added calcium; added vitamins
SoGood	Added calcium and vitamins; chilled and longlife
Sojasun	Calcium-enriched soya milk with live cultures
Suma Wholefoods	Soya milk powder
Sunrise (Soya Health Foods)	Sweetened and unsweetened soya drinks
supermarkets	Own-brand sweetened and unsweetened, with added calcium
Unisoy Gold	Soya milk with added calcium

Generally, organic soya milks have no calcium or vitamins added, and 'value' brands don't either. Choose carefully and try lots of different varieties until you get one to suit your taste.

Other dairy-free milks

Blue Dragon Foods	Tinned coconut milk; fat-reduced coconut milk
Darifree	Selection of potato milks
Ecomil	Quinoa drink; almond drink; hazelnut drink; instant almond drink powder; organic almond and soya drink
First Foods	Oat drink: calcium-enriched
Oatly	Oat drink: vanilla, chocolate, added calcium
Plamil Foods	*White Sun* – pea protein alternative to milk: sweetened, unsweetened
Probios	Rice drink with added calcium, organic
Provamel	Rice drink: with or without calcium and vitamins
Rice Dream	Rice drink: organic original, vanilla, chocolate, carob, calcium-enriched. Range includes lunchbox size: original, chocolate, vanilla; 200ml and 1 litre sizes
Tiger White	Chufa milk: sweetened and unsweetened
Vitariz	Organic rice drink

Dairy-free creams

AlproSoya	Soya single cream
Blue Dragon Foods	Creamed coconut
Brooklyn Foods	*Smackin' Good* whip topping ('squirty cream') (available in kosher shops)
First Foods	Oat 'Supreme' cream
Granovita	*Cremovita* organic soya whipping cream
Granose (Haldane Foods)	Longlife soya cream
Oatly	*Cuisine* 'cream'
Rich's	Whip topping
Snowcrest	*Big Top* Parev cream whip (from kosher shops)
SoGood	UHT soya cream
Sojami Organic Supplies	Dairy-free soya-based vegan crème fraîche

Cheese and cheese spreads

Anglesey Foods	Cheese spreads: coriander & lemon, plain, garlic & herb; hard cheeses; *Vegerella Biddy Merkins* cheese substitute – Italian/Mexican
Bute Island Foods	*Scheese* (hard 'cheese'): cheddar, cheddar with chives, cheshire, edam, gouda, hickory cheddar, mozzarella, stilton, emmental, blue
Free & Easy	Cheese-flavour sauce mix
Galaxy Foods	Soya cheese slices: cheddar, mozzarella. ***Beware of rice cheese slices***, as they contain casein
Kallo Foods	*Fromsoya* soya cheese spreads: original, garlic, onion, parsley
MH Ltd	*Florentino Parmazzano* a non-animal dairy-free parmesan style
Redwood	*Cheezly* tofu cheese – red cheddar, white cheddar, bar-b-q style, garlic & parsley, pizza style, mozzarella, edam; slices; melting blocks
Tofutti	Cream cheese: French onion, plain, garlic & herbs, chives & herbs, country vegetable

Note that several other soya cheeses of US origin (e.g. Rice Parmesan, Light & Less, Rice Slice and Soya Kaas) are designed for the low-fat market rather than the dairy-free market. As a result, to improve their consistency they include *casein* – which is a milk protein – making them unsuitable for a dairy-free diet.

'Cheese' flavouring

Nutritional yeast-flakes are a product made from molasses and produced specifically for the healthfood market. It is a yellow flake with a sweet cheesy taste, and is excellent as flavouring for cheese-type sauces. It can also be used as a topping sprinkled on lasagne or pizza or mixed with mashed potato and cooked in the oven as cheese and potato bake. The flakes can also be mixed with a dairy-free margarine to be spread on bread and toasted under the grill.

Engevita Nutritional Flakes from Marigold Healthfoods are available from most healthfood shops. Alternatively, *The Uncheese Cookbook* (Stepaniak, see Appendix 3) contains recipes for you to make your own dairy-free cheese.

Dairy-free pesto

G Costa & Co. Ltd	*Zest Foods*: vegan pesto; sun-dried tomato paste
Meridian	Green pesto; red pesto
Suma	Vegan pesto

Margarine/Fat

Windmill Organics	*Biona*: extra virgin olive oil organic dairy-free spread; soya-free; dairy-free; vegan Organic sunflower vegetable spread free from dairy/milk products and their derivatives; vegan
Flora	White Flora
Granose (Haldane Foods)	Soya margarine; sunflower margarine; diet half-fat spread; olive grove margarine; low-salt vegetable margarine
Granovita	Non-hydrogenated sunflower margarine; non-hydrogenated low-fat spread
Matthews Foods	*Pure*: sunflower margarine; soya spread
Meridian Foods	Soya margarine
Rakusen's	*Tomor*: block margarine; sunflower tubs
Smilde Food Group	Sunflower spread
Suma Wholefoods	Low-fat spread; soya spread; 100% sunflower spread; organic spread
supermarkets	Own-brands of soya margarines; dairy-free low-fat spreads
Vitaquel	Margarine selection: organic; extra; cuisine; low fat

Dairy-free yoghurts

Alpro Soya	500ml: forest fruits, plain. 4x125ml: strawberry, peach, black cherry, red cherry, peach & mango, raspberry & vanilla OY smooth 4x125ml: strawberry & banana, peach & pear
Granose	Soya yoghurts: apricot, blackcurrant & apple, peach melba, strawberry
Granovita	*Deluxe Soyage* – non-dairy cultured soya dessert: peach & apricot, raspberry, strawberry, natural, black cherry, banana, mango, tropical *Soyage Organic*: strawberry, peach, forest fruits
SoGood	Natural, peach & passion fruit, black cherry, strawberry, pineapple
Sojasun	Natural, apricot & guava, raspberry & passion fruit. Live yoghurts
Unisoy	Raspberry, black cherry, peach melba

Sauces

Meridian	White wine & mushroom, korma, mushroom, sun-dried tomato, tikka masala, tomato & herb, pepper & mushroom
Safetoeat	Chinese, curry, Italian, tomato and many other flavours
Sauces of Choice	Selection of dairy-free curry sauces, cook-in sauces, condiments and dressings

Non-frozen desserts

Alpro Soya	Organic soya desserts: cartons of custard; vanilla, chocolate
	Pots: vanilla, chocolate, forest fruits, caramel
Probios	Rice dessert: vanilla, chocolate
Sojasun	Non-dairy dessert: strawberry, raspberry & passion fruit, lemon. All organic

Ice-creams

Fayrefield Foods	*Swedish Glace* – 1 litre: strawberry, raspberry, vanilla, chocolate, mocha, caramel; raspberry cones
First Foods	Oat-based dairy-free ice-cream: Cornish block, 'Supreme' choc on a stick
Soya Health Foods Ltd	*Sunrise* soya-based carob choc-ice
Tofutti	Individual tubs: vanilla fudge
	Cones: vanilla & pecan nut
	Ice-cream cake: 'Rock 'n' Roll' (similar to Viennetta)
	Fudge lollies
	Organic ice-creams: vanilla, chocolate, strawberry, mango & passion fruit
Turtle Mountain	Ice-cream: vanilla, cookie avalanche, chocolate obsession, mint, chocolate brownie

Chocolate spreads

Chocoreal	Three types of organic chocolate spreads
Plamil Foods	Chocolate, chocolate orange – organic

Chocolate

AllergyCare	*Whizzers*: chocolate beans; chocolate footballs; speckled eggs
Animal Aid	Huge selection of non-dairy boxes and bars of dairy-free chocolate and fudge
Buxton Foods	*The Stamp Collection* – dairy-free chocolates: sultana, apricot, sunflower seed, Easter bunny
Devon Fudge Direct	Chocolate flavoured
Doves Farm	Chocolate chip cookies; plain chocolate digestives
Dr Hadwen Trust	Selection of handmade non-dairy vegan chocolates: chocolate Brazils; cherry liqueurs; assortments; mint creams; chocolate ginger; gold selection; chocolate animals; etc.
Humdinger Ltd	Dairy-free chocolate bars: rice crisp, tangerine, roasted almond, original
Kinnerton	Bars of dark chocolate and other confectionery, including seasonal items such as advent calendars and Easter eggs, guaranteed free from nut, egg, gluten and dairy
Lyme Regis Foods	Chocolate marzipan bar
Plamil Foods	*Expressions* non-dairy milk chocolate: organic dark, organic orange, organic mint dark
	Non-dairy carob bars: plain, hazelnut, orange; no added sugar; no added sugar drops
	Martello non-dairy milk chocolate: dark plain, hazelnut, mint
	Dairy-free milk chocolate
Rapunzel	Swiss chocolate: plain organic, plain with almonds organic
Shepherd Boy	*Just So* carob bars: crispy, orange, peppermint, ginger
Suma	Carob drops
supermarkets	Own-brands. Various – see their 'free from' lists
Tropical Source	Chocolate bars: toasted almond, hazelnut, rice crisp, raspberry, mint, rich dark
	Production line guaranteed dairy-free
Vegan Society	Fine mint chocolates; organic gourmet chocolate truffles
Viva!	Selection of dairy-free bars and boxes of chocolates
Whole Earth Foods	*Green & Black* organic dairy-free chocolate: organic dark, Maya gold

Remember, too, that kosher foods are dairy-free.

Chocolate on a dairy-free diet

Allergic reactions have been reported after eating chocolate listed as milk-free on a 'free from' list and on the product label and with no mention of any milk derivatives in the list of ingredients. On investigation it has become apparent that these reactions were not because the chocolate contained milk in the ingredients but because it had traces of milk from the production line during manufacture. (Learn more about cross-contamination in Chapter 15.)

Production lines used for chocolate are notoriously difficult to clean because of the high fat content and the nature of the product.

A way around this is to eat only chocolate that is made on a production line that is never used for products containing milk. Kinnerton, Humdinger and Plamil (vegan products only) are three examples of manufacturers whose factories do this.

Alternatively, phone the company to see how they can back up their dairy-free claim. Ask if they routinely test their chocolate for the presence of milk, and whether other products containing milk are made on that production line. An informed choice will then, hopefully, be a safer choice.

EGG-FREE DIET

EGG ALLERGY

Egg allergy is much more common in children than in adults. However, around 85% of children with egg allergy will grow out of it by the age of 5.

It is not uncommon for well-cooked egg such as that found in cake to be tolerated but less-well-cooked eggs such as scrambled or fried eggs, omelettes and pancakes to cause allergic reactions in the same individual. This is because cooking 'denatures' (changes the form of) the proteins that cause reactions, making them less allergenic.

Because of the good chance that they will grow out of egg allergy, affected children are often offered testing at an allergy clinic to check whether they have grown out of it. This may be offered yearly until the age of 7 or 8; after this age they are less likely to grow out of the allergy although many do go on to do so.

If you are allergic to hen's eggs, you should avoid eggs from all birds because the proteins are very similar.

Is it safe to eat chicken and other poultry?

Yes! This is because the proteins in the flesh are different from the (allergenic) proteins in eggs.

People with egg allergy who also have a poultry allergy, should of course avoid it. However, if you are tolerating chicken and other poultry and wish to eat it, you can continue to do so.

FOODS CONTAINING EGGS

It is relatively easy to avoid obvious sources of eggs such as boiled, scrambled, omelettes and quiche. In the EU any packaged manufactured food must tell you on the label if it contains egg. Foods sold loose and foods other people have prepared do not list the ingredients and may well contain 'hidden' egg. Furthermore, foods sold outside the EU are not governed by the same food-labelling laws, so they could contain undeclared egg; they might also have egg derivatives 'hidden' under any of the following names on the label:

Albumen	Egg yolk	Ovoglobulin
Dried egg	Frozen egg	Ovomucin
Egg (all bird eggs)	Globulin	Ovovitellin
Egg powder	Lecithin (E322)*	Pasteurised egg
Egg protein	Livetin	Vitellin
Egg white	Ovalbumin	

(*Theoretically, lecithin can be derived from egg, but in practice this is rare; it is usually soya-based. However, some studies suggest that egg lecithin does not in fact trigger a reaction. In the EU the source of the lecithin must be declared.)

Table 10.4 has examples of foods that contain egg that is well cooked, loosely cooked and raw.

Living safely on an egg-free diet

- Always read the food ingredient label to see if it contains egg (in any form). If the food does not have a label – such as bakery goods – *do not* eat it. (See Chapter 9 for information about how to understand and read food labels.)
- Understand cross-contamination issues (see Chapter 15).

Table 10.4 Classification of food containing egg

Well-cooked egg	Loosely cooked egg	Raw egg
Cakes	Pancakes	Fresh mousse
Biscuits	Meringues	Fresh mayonnaise
Dried egg pasta	Lemon curd	Fresh ice-cream
Egg in sausages or prepared meat dishes	Quiche	Fresh sorbet
	Scrambled egg	Royal icing
Well-cooked fresh egg pasta	Boiled egg	Horseradish sauce
	Fried egg	Tartar sauce
Egg glaze on pastry	Omelette	Raw egg in cake mix (tasted before baking!) and other uncooked dishes
	Poached egg	
	Egg in batter	
	Egg in breadcrumbs	
	Hollandaise sauce	

- Eat only foods that you are completely sure are safe to eat.
- To add variety to your diet when you cannot eat eggs you can use existing recipes, but with whole egg replacer instead of whole egg, and egg white replacer instead of egg white. (Some common replacements for egg are listed at the end of this section.)
- Substitute eggs with something else, depending on their purpose in the recipe: leavening agent, raising agent, glazing agent, binding agent, source of liquid. Table 10.5 shows alternatives, according to the usual function of the egg in the recipe.
- Try some recipes that are egg-free. These may be recipes that just happen to be egg-free or they may be from a vegan or special-diet cookbook (see Appendix 3), or those supplied with the egg replacer.
- Request a 'free from egg' list from the supermarket(s) where you shop. This is a list of all their own-brand products that are free from egg. It is a free service, but you may have to ask the supermarket's head office for the list.
- Request a 'free from egg' list from your favourite manufacturers (e.g. Walkers, Findus).
- Make use of foods manufactured specifically for people allergic to eggs (e.g. egg-free mayonnaise and egg-free cakes).
- Buy vegan foods, as they are always egg-free.

- Eat out in a vegan restaurant or go to a vegan guesthouse or one that caters specifically for special diets. As well as enjoying the treat, it will allow you access to lots of other recipe ideas; you may be able to chat to the chef and look at his or her cookbook selection if you ask nicely!

Tales of the un*egg*spected . . .

Below are examples of items that you might never have guessed could contain egg:

- some medicines,
- freshly made consommé soup (egg may be used as a clarifier),
- hair shampoo and conditioner,
- royal icing and icing flowers,
- nutritional supplements (e.g. vitamin and mineral preparations),
- pet foods,
- some wines and champagnes (egg albumen can be used as a clarifying agent),
- vaccinations grown on an egg culture (discuss this with your doctor).

Table 10.5 Egg substitutes

Purpose of egg in recipe	Substitute
Leavening	15ml (1 tbsp) baking powder + 30ml (2 tbsp) liquid
Glazing	Sugar and water or gelatine glaze
Binding	Soya milk; soya dessert; custard; mashed banana; soya cream; white sauce
(1 egg =)	50g (1¾ oz) tofu; *or* 100ml (⅓ cup) water + 5ml (1 tsp) arrowroot powder + 10ml (2 tsp) guar gum
Liquid (1 egg =)	100ml (⅓ cup) apple juice; 15ml (1 tbsp) vinegar; 60ml (4 tbsp) pureed apricot
Raising agent (1 egg =)	15ml (1 tbsp) baking powder; 3.75ml (¾ tsp) bicarbonate of soda + 10ml (2 tsp) cider vinegar

Note Remember that any alcoholic drinks over 1.2% proof must, by law, declare if the product contains egg, however small the amount. The Vegan Society and most supermarkets selling own-brands can provide a list of wines and champagnes that have not been clarified with egg. Alternatively, buy from a vegan wine merchant. Vintage Roots Ltd is a major independent merchant in the UK selling vegan wine direct to customers by mail order and to shops and restaurants (contact details in Appendix 1). Healthfood shops are another source of vegan wines.

VACCINES

Measles, mumps and rubella (MMR) vaccine
It is very important that you do not prevent your child from having the MMR vaccination. The risks from these three diseases are much greater than the minute risk of your child having an allergic reaction.

The MMR and the influenza vaccines *may* be cultured on chick embryo cells, but it is unlikely that the vaccine is contaminated by egg protein. It is extremely unlikely that this vaccine could then cause a reaction in an egg-allergic individual but make sure that the doctor knows about your child's allergy so that he can advise you accordingly.

Yellow fever and influenza vaccines
If you have a severe egg allergy, you should avoid yellow fever and flu vaccines.

ALTERNATIVES FOR EGGS

Substitute for	Name of product	Made by
Whole egg	Whole Egg Replacer	Allergycare
	Ener-G Egg Replacer	General Dietary
	Loprofin Egg Replacer	SHS
Egg white	Rite-Diet Egg White Replacer	SHS
Egg yolk, egg white, or whole egg	No-Egg Replacer	Orgran

Whole egg replacers are available on prescription or to buy. Egg white replacers are available only from pharmacists.

EGG-FREE FOODS

Allergycare	Egg-free omelette mix (contains dairy)
Avalon	Egg-free dip and salad dressing: plain, garlic, cajun
Blue Dragon	Egg-free whole-wheat noodles and rice noodles
Clearspring	Egg-free wheat noodles; egg-free wheat-free noodles
G Costa & Co. Ltd	*Zest Foods* Vegan pesto and vegan gluten-free pesto
Granovita	Egg-free mayonnaise: plain, lemon, garlic
manufacturers	Obtain their 'free from' list so that you can identify their egg-free products
Mrs Crimble's	Dutch apple cake free from egg, wheat and dairy
Orgran	Sponge pudding mixes: chocolate; lemon
(Community Foods)	Pancake mix
Plamil	Egg-free mayonnaise: garlic, plain, tarragon, plain organic, lemon grass
Suma	Vegannaise: plain, garlic. Vegan pesto: red, green
Sunnyvale	Banana cake; ginger cake; fruit cake; malt loaf
supermarkets	Own-brands: obtain their 'free from' lists so that their egg-free products can be identified
Village Bakery	Egg-free slices: date, apricot
	Cakes: fruit cake
	Fruit bars: nut; seed; fruit

PEANUT-FREE AND NUT-FREE DIETS

There has been a lot of publicity about peanut and nut allergies in recent years. This is because these allergies are becoming more common and also because a number of deaths related to peanut and nut allergy have been reported in the mass media.

Peanuts and nuts are often talked about as one and the same thing. They do not, however, belong to the same food family. Peanuts are legumes, which grow in the ground – so they are also known as groundnuts. They are from the *Leguminosae* plant family, which contains over 30 species, including peas, beans, lentils, soya beans, carob and liquorice. (For information about food families, see Chapter 12.) Some people who are allergic to peanuts are concerned that they may also be allergic to these other foods in this family. A report from the USA found that 5% of the children studied who had reacted to one legume had symptoms with multiple legumes. Nevertheless, if you are allergic to peanuts it is unnecessary to eliminate other legumes (such as peas, beans and lentils) from your diet unless there is good reason to suspect that they cause problems.

Botanically, peanuts are unrelated to tree nuts such as Brazil, macadamia, cashew, almond, walnut, pecan, pistachio and hazelnut. However, it is fairly common for someone with peanut allergy to react to these as well. Whether you should avoid all nuts because you are allergic to peanuts, and vice-versa, is an important question. *Some people with peanut allergy can eat tree nuts without a problem* – allergy tests may help to determine this. If you have lived safely for many years without taking these precautionary measures, you could – in theory – continue to do so but you will be taking a risk (perhaps you have just been lucky so far). It is generally recommended that you exclude all peanuts and all tree nuts from your diet. The reasons for this are:

- cross-contamination;
- adulteration – one nut type or peanut is disguised as another; for example, peanuts re-formed into an almond shape or crushed and added to a curry with almond essence as a cheap alternative to ground almonds;
- you may go on to develop an allergy to other nuts, as some studies have shown.

OTHER NAMES FOR PEANUT

As well as the Latin name, *Arachis hypogaea*, peanuts have several other English names:

earth nut	groundnut	monkey-nut
goober nuts	mandalona nut	pinda
goober peas	manilla nut	pinder

You can look up the names in other languages in a comprehensive dictionary, but don't assume you can correctly pronounce or understand the word when it is spoken. Alternatively, contact Allergy UK for a translation in most languages. See also the translation section at the end of this chapter.

PEANUT DERIVATIVES

Peanut derivatives in pre-packaged manufactured foods for sale in the EU must, by law, be labelled as 'peanut'. They include:

- arachis (peanut) oil (see below),
- peanut flour,
- peanut protein,
- unrefined peanut oil (see below).

Some sources of hydrolysed vegetable protein are derived from peanuts.

PEANUT OIL

Peanut oil is also known as groundnut oil and arachis oil. It may be refined or unrefined.

The Seed Crushers and Oil Processors Association (SCOPA), of which all UK refiners of edible oil are members, funded research into the allergenicity of peanut oil. Its findings were published in 1997 in the *British Medical Journal*. The report concluded that **refined** peanut oil poses little or no risk to people with peanut allergy; in the unlikely event of a reaction, it would almost certainly be mild. **Unrefined** (crude) peanut oil should be avoided, because it may contain minute traces of peanut protein.

By law, pre-packaged foods manufactured for sale in the EU must include in the ingredients list any refined and unrefined peanut oils used in the product.

OTHER NUT ALLERGIES

Other nut allergies are common. The 'culprit' nuts are common in the following foods:

Almonds

almond yoghurt	ice-cream dishes and toppings
Bakewell tart	Indian dishes (e.g. peshwari and korma)
biscuits	marzipan
Chinese dishes	mincemeat
Danish pastries	nougat
flourless cake	soups

Cashew nuts

Chinese dishes (e.g. kung po and chow mein)
Indian dishes (e.g. tikka, pasanda, masalla and Bombay mix)
pesto sauce
Thai dishes (e.g. satay)

Hazelnuts

breakfast cereals (e.g. muesli, crunchynut cornflakes)
chocolate bars (e.g. Topic)
chocolate spread with nuts
chocolates, especially truffles and praline
Indian dishes (e.g. Bombay mix)
ice-cream toppings
Malaysian and Indonesian dishes (e.g. bang-bang)
paté
peanut-flavour jellybeans
pie bases
prepared rice dishes
prepared salads
savoury snacks
stuffings
Thai dishes (e.g. satay)
vegetarian foods (e.g. nut burgers and nut loaf)
yoghurts with muesli or nuts

Other nuts and mixed nuts

Brazil nuts in chocolates or mincemeat
chestnut stuffing
chocolates, toffees in bars or boxes (e.g. pralines, truffles)
coronation sauces
fruit cakes, festive puddings, mince pies
ice-cream and toppings
macadamia nuts
paté
peanut-flavour jellybeans
pecan nuts; pecan pie
pie bases
pistachio nuts
prepared rice dishes
prepared salads
soy sauces
vegetarian foods (e.g. nut burgers and sausages)
walnuts (e.g. Waldorf salad, cakes, Walnut Whip)

By law, pre-packaged foods sold in the EU must state clearly on the label if they contain any nuts.

'MAY CONTAIN' WARNINGS ON FOOD LABELS

Food manufacturers and retailers have become increasingly allergy-aware over the past few years. They are striving to ensure that the public is informed about the food they eat. Because of cross-contamination issues (see Chapter 15) and possible litigation, 'may contain' warnings have now been placed on many foods that do not contain peanuts or nuts but may have become contaminated with traces of these foods. This has caused a lot of discontent among people with a peanut or nut allergy, because it has resulted in a vast restriction on food choices. Nevertheless, if you ignore 'may contain' labelling, you are taking an unmeasurable risk.

IS PEANUT OR NUT ALLERGY ON THE INCREASE?

Peanuts are now one of the main causes of food allergy reactions in the UK. Allergy clinics report an increase in the number of patients with peanut allergy, particularly in children. The exact reason for this is not known but it is suspected that a number of factors are involved (see Chapter 1). A major factor is the increased availability of peanuts in the British diet. This has led to increased exposure of babies (both in the womb and during breast-feeding) and young children to peanuts and peanut products and their proteins. Because the immune system (see Chapter 1) is not fully developed this early in life, such exposure may be one of the causes of the increased prevalence of nut and peanut allergies. More research is needed to determine whether this is true.

HOW DANGEROUS IS PEANUT/NUT ALLERGY?

Fatalities due to peanut and nut allergies are rare. Reported cases are more common in young people in their late teens and early twenties, particularly when they eat outside the home. This may be because they become more independent and are no longer protected by their parents. Perhaps some rebel against having to carry their adrenaline everywhere they go. Maybe alcohol consumption is a factor – less care is taken and the early signs of a reaction are missed?

We know that the risk of having a severe allergic reaction is increased in people with asthma, so improving asthma control with correct treatment is a good starting point.

There are many positive ways in which you can deal with these issues. The Anaphylaxis Campaign has a comprehensive booklet, aimed specifically at this age group, on how the risks can be minimised; it also runs youth workshops and parent workshops.

REDUCING THE DANGER OF A SEVERE REACTION

Outgrowing the allergy

It is thought that 10–20% of people (usually children) do outgrow a nut/peanut allergy. However, it is impossible to predict who will lose their allergy, and you should *never* try to test yourself. You should be properly assessed with skin-prick and RAST testing and then, if appropriate, with a carefully monitored 'oral challenge' (see also Chapter 2, 'Food Allergy Tests'). Get medical advice about this.

Desensitisation

Desensitisation is unsuitable for someone with a severe food allergy.

Vaccination

Vaccination against nut/peanut allergy is not currently available.

Airline travel and nuts

The problems caused by nuts during air travel are discussed in Chapter 16 ('Holidays and Travelling').

Nut allergies and schools

See Chapter 6 for coping with food allergies when at school.

EATING OUT WITH A PEANUT/NUT ALLERGY

If you have a severe peanut/nut allergy and you want to eat out, you must be vigilant, ask all the right questions and, of course, carry your medication. Unless you have prepared the food yourself, you cannot be sure that it is completely safe.

If you decide that you are prepared to take this risk, the following suggestions will help to keep it to a minimum:

- Avoid Chinese, Thai, Malaysian and Indian restaurants. They use a lot of nuts and peanuts in their dishes, so there is a risk of cross-contamination (see Chapter 15).

- Use the same restaurant regularly, so that the staff become familiar with your needs.
- Go at a quiet time rather than when things are hectic and your needs might be unintentionally overlooked.
- Patronise a place that has a nut/peanut policy and general allergy-awareness.
- Give the chef written guidelines about your needs, to prevent ambiguity. Ask that they be placed in a file for future use, or take a copy to the chef every time you are planning to eat in that restaurant or café.
- Choose simple dishes that are less likely to be contaminated.
- Telephone first, so that your meal can be made in advance and covered, ready to heat up later when the kitchen is busy.
- If you are not confident that your needs can be met but would like to join friends or colleagues who are eating out, ask if you can take your own ready-prepared food that can be heated up (or take a cold dish) and brought to you alongside the others' meals. Most places are more than happy for you to do this rather than risk taking responsibility for your food! (See also Chapter 14, 'Eating Away from Home'.)

Tales of the un*nut*spected!
Besides being a source of human nutrition, peanut and peanut products are used in animal and bird feeds and in skin creams. Under the European Union Cosmetic Directive, which came into force in December 1997, cosmetics products containing peanut oil must list the ingredients. The name used is usually *Arachis hypogaea*. (See Chapter 9, 'Food Labelling', for more details.)

Traces of nuts and cross-contamination
Traces of peanuts or peanut dust can be inhaled when you are near someone who is eating them – such as where peanut snacks are distributed with drinks – or where a large number of nuts are on display – as in a supermarket at Christmas time. Cross-contamination can also occur, and is discussed in Chapter 15.

MISTAKEN PEANUT DERIVATIVES

Carob This is a member of the legume family. Research suggests that carob is safe for people with peanut/nut allergy.

Coconut and nutmeg Despite the word 'nut' in their names, coconut and nutmeg are not related to peanuts or nuts. An allergic reaction to either is unlikely but has been known to occur in a small number of individuals, including people with nut/peanut allergy. If you are concerned, NHS allergy clinics may do an allergy test if you ask for one.

E471 and E472 These are food additives that act as emulsifiers. It is technically possible, though highly unlikely, for E471 and E472 to be derived from peanut oil. Even if peanut oil was the source, the risk of an allergic reaction would be extremely low because the oil would have been refined. If they *are* derived from peanut oil and are present in food sold in the EU, the label must tell you this.

Essence of nuts Although there have been no reported reactions to essence of nuts such as almond essence, you are advised to avoid them.

Lecithin Lecithin is an emulsifier, usually derived from unrefined soya oil or, very occasionally, from egg. SCOPA (see earlier in this chapter) has stated 'Lecithin is not derived from peanut oil'.

Palm nuts and pine nuts Palm nuts and pine nuts are not botanically related to peanuts or tree nuts. As with any foods, though, they may cause reactions in a small number of people who are not necessarily allergic to peanuts or nuts.

ALTERNATIVE PEANUT/NUT-FREE TREATS

Peanut/nut-free chocolates

It's Nut Free	Selection of flapjacks, muffins, brownies, shortbread, cakes
Kinnerton	Good range of peanut/nut-free chocolate made in the UK on a production line separate from their peanut/nut varieties
Nestlé	Selection of peanut/nut-free chocolate, including Easter, Christmas and novelty varieties

Peanut/nut-free sweets

Sweets are easy to locate. Any 'free from' list will help you, and most packets are well labelled.

Bakery goods

Fabulous Bakin' Boys	Flapjacks, cupcakes and other sweet treats

LUPIN ALLERGY

Lupin allergy has been recognised for some time in Europe, where lupin flour is used widely to replace cereal grains in rice, pasta and bakery products. The major allergens in lupin are also found in peanuts, so people who are allergic to peanuts may also be allergic to lupin because of cross-reactivity of these allergens.

Because lupin flour is used widely in mainland Europe, you should be careful when staying there or eating products brought back from there.

By the end of 2007, lupin will be one of 14 foods that must be labelled on pre-packaged manufactured foods for sale within the EU.

SESAME-FREE DIET

SESAME SEED ALLERGY

Sesame seeds are becoming increasingly popular in the UK. Also increasing is the small but significant number of people who are severely allergic to them. If you are allergic to sesame, you must avoid it completely – both in its cooked and in its uncooked form.

Sesame seeds are used extensively in the food industry, so it is important to read food labels carefully. By law, sesame must be labelled on pre-packed manufactured foods sold in the EU. Sesame can also be known as:

- anjoli/anjonjoli
- benne seeds/benne oil
- gingili/gingelly
- oleum
- *Sesamum indicum*
- simsim
- teel
- til

Sesamum indicum is the Latin name for sesame, and has been used in labelling on cosmetics, toiletries and perfumes since 1998. (See also Chapter 9 for more about food labelling.)

SESAME OIL

Sesame oil made from pulped ('cold pressing') sesame seeds is one of the few oils that is usually used without being refined. This unrefined oil is likely to contain a significant amount of sesame seed protein, the part of the seed that can trigger an allergic reaction. If you have a sesame allergy, you must avoid all forms of sesame oil.

Because sesame seeds are very small, they are easily transferred by cross-contamination (see Chapter 15).

YOU SHOULD KNOW

- Unwrapped bakery goods may be contaminated with sesame seeds from other products, so only buy bakery products if they are pre-wrapped.
- Sesame seeds often contaminate delicatessen counters, so it is unsafe to buy from a delicatessen. Most delicatessen products are also available pre-packed, so you can buy these instead.
- 'Mixed spices' contain various spice seeds that may include sesame, so always check the ingredients label thoroughly.
- Most food manufacturers and supermarkets provide a 'free from sesame' list of their own-brand products (see Chapter 13, 'Eating In'). This will help you to choose suitable food to buy for a sesame-free diet.
- Sesame is used in some cosmetics. Since the passage of the Cosmetic Labelling Act in 1998, its inclusion must be listed among the ingredients.
- Sesame is sometimes used in medical preparations such as plasters, liniments, ointments and soaps. Always check the ingredients listings.
- Sesame oil may occasionally be present in medicines. Always ask your pharmacist to check any medication that you are planning to take.
- Sesame contains two natural antioxidants: sesamol and sesamoline. They both retain their properties during frying at high temperatures, which is why sesame oil is so highly prized by Chinese and Japanese chefs, who use it in many dishes. If you have a severe allergy to sesame, you should therefore avoid Chinese and Japanese cuisine.

Eating food that you have not prepared *yourself* carries the greatest risk of triggering a life-threatening anaphylactic reaction. This is partly because of the risks from cross-contamination (see Chapter 15) and partly because you might not recognise a dish as containing sesame if it is written in a language that is unfamiliar to you. Eating out requires a great deal of caution. The following are examples of foods that may lead to anaphylaxis because they include sesame:

- bread, biscuits and crackers,
- soups,
- mixed salads, salad dressings,
- vegetable burgers,
- sauces, marinades, stir-fry sauces,
- desserts,
- Chinese, Japanese, Greek, Mexican and Lebanese restaurant meals,
- humous, tahini and halva.

Humous is high on the list for triggering an allergic reaction, as are tahini and halva.

For more general advice on eating safely with a severe food allergy, see also Chapter 9 ('Food Labelling'), Chapter 13 ('Eating In') and Chapter 16 ('Eating Away from Home').

SHELLFISH-FREE AND FISH-FREE DIETS

As concerns about dietary fat and cholesterol have increased, seafood (shellfish) and fish (especially oily fish) have become a more prominent part of our diet. They can be eaten as a snack, sandwich filler, starter or main meal and are cooked in a variety of ways. Sushi, which is a raw fish delicacy, is also very fashionable.

FISH-FREE DIET

If you react to one type of fish, you are usually advised to avoid all fish because of the risk of cross-contamination in markets, restaurants and fish counters. There is also cross-reactivity because all fish contain the same main allergenic protein called parvalbumin – if you are allergic to one type of fish, you will often react to other types.

Unlike most allergenic foods, the vapours of fish cooking can trigger allergic reactions in some very sensitive people. If this is you. take care when eating out and when passing an open fish counter or a fish and chip shop.

Eating out

In restaurants, be sure to inform staff that you have a fish allergy, as they may use oil to fry fish and then fry your food in it. The ingredients of all stocks and soups and other foods and sauces that may contain fish extract should be checked. To prevent cross-contamination and to ensure that your meal is definitely fish-free, or if you are affected by cooking vapours, choose a vegetarian or vegan restaurant.

Dishes that contain fish include:

- paella,
- bouillabaisse,
- gumbo (creole dish from Louisiana),
- frito misto (Mediterranean dish),
- fruits de mer (French),
- surimi (often in pizza).
- Caesar salad usually contains anchovies,
- caponata (Sicilian relish),
- fish sauce is a common ingredient used instead of salt in Eastern cooking,
- patum peperium (Gentleman's Relish) is a spread made with anchovies,
- Worcestershire sauce contains anchovies.

Food legislation requires any manufactured pre-packaged foods sold in the EU to clearly label the presence of fish on the ingredients list.

'HIDDEN' FISH

- **Anchovy**, which is a small fish in the herring family, is often used as a flavour enhancer in Worcestershire sauce.
- **Aspic** is a savoury jelly, used as a glazing agent, that may be derived from fish.
- **Caviar** is the roe of the sturgeon and other fish; it may be used as a relish or garnish.
- **Cod liver oil** is the oil extracted from the liver of the cod and related fish, and is often used as a nutritional supplement.

- **Vitamin D₃** (cholecalciferol) may be derived from fish oil, for use as a nutritional supplement.

Tales of the un*fish*spected

Fish and their derivatives can sometimes be an ingredient of the following:

- cosmetics, toiletries, soaps (see also Chapter 9, 'Food Labelling'),
- glues and adhesives,
- nutritional supplements (e.g. vitamins),
- pet foods, including fish food,

The list above is just for your information. Even if you are allergic to fish, this does not mean that you will be allergic to these products. But if you are having a reaction and don't know why, one of these products might be the answer. Please discuss the matter with your allergy specialist.

To avoid fish successfully, use products recommended by the Vegetarian Society and the Vegan Society. The Vegan Society lists suitable products in its handbook, *The Animal-Free Shopper* (edited by Bird, Farhall, Rofe and Whitlock; see Appendix 3 for details).

SHELLFISH-FREE DIET

A shellfish allergy is an abnormal response of the body to the proteins found in shellfish. In order to avoid manufactured foods that contain shellfish ingredients, it is important to read food labels. By law, any pre-packaged manufactured food must clearly label the presence of crustaceans but molluscs will not have to be labelled until the end of 2007.

Crustaceans

- crab (crabsticks)
- lobster, langouste, langoustine, scampi, coral, tomalley
- crawfish, crayfish, ecrevisse, abalone
- shrimp, prawns, crevette

Molluscs

- *Bivalves*: mussels, oysters, scallops, clam (cherrystone, littleneck, pismo, quahog)

- *Gastropods*: cockle, periwinkle, sea urchin, limpet, snails
- *Cephalopods*: squid, cuttlefish, octopus

Some of the names listed above may not be familiar to you but they are included because you may come across them when you go abroad or eat in restaurants.

Someone who reacts to one type of shellfish is usually advised to avoid all other shellfish because of the risk of cross-contamination. This is particularly an issue in restaurants and fish counters, where there is a high risk of cross-contamination occurring.

Shellfish shell and skeleton derivatives
Although it is the flesh of the shellfish that contains the allergen, people with shellfish allergy are advised to avoid shellfish shells and skeletons. Glucosamine, used in the treatment of osteoarthritis, is derived from the skeletons of shellfish (usually shrimps). Some recent evidence suggests that it is tolerated by people with shellfish allergy but it may be safer to choose a vegetarian or vegan supplement. Chondroitin is a suitable alternative.

Some nutritional supplement tablets may contain ground shellfish, so either check with the manufacturer or choose a vegetarian- or vegan-approved product. Whether these supplements will cause allergic symptoms if consumed is unclear, but it is best to play safe.

SCROMBOID POISONING

Scromboid poisoning occurs after eating certain fish that contain high levels of histadine, such as tuna, mackerel and sardines. When they are not refrigerated and start to 'go off' the histadine converts to histamine, leading to scromboid poisoning. The symptoms resemble an allergic reaction and usually occur within minutes to an hour after eating the fish. As a result, sufferers think they are allergic to fish, when in fact they are experiencing a scromboid poisoning reaction. They are not allergic to fish and will not have to avoid fish in the future.

WHEAT-FREE AND GLUTEN-FREE DIETS

Gluten is a protein found in wheat, rye, barley and oats. Ingredients to be avoided on food labels are these four grains, in all their various forms. Although oats do contain gluten, some people who are unable to tolerate gluten from other cereals are able to tolerate oats. Be sure to discuss with your doctor whether you can include oats in your diet.

WHAT IS THE DIFFERENCE BETWEEN WHEAT-FREE AND GLUTEN-FREE?

- **Wheat-free** means something that is free from wheat only.
- **Gluten-free** means something that is free from gluten – which can be found in barley, rye and oats as well as wheat. All of these *can* be eaten on a gluten-free diet if the gluten has been removed from them. The most common example of this is *de-glutenised wheat*: because the gluten has been removed, it is quite safe for it to be eaten on a gluten-free diet. (However, it is *not* safe for a wheat-free diet.)

AVOIDING WHEAT

It is very difficult to avoid eating wheat, because:

- wheat is one of the staple foods of the British diet (e.g. bread, cakes, biscuits, pizza, pasta – the last usually made of durum wheat),
- wheat is present in a great many manufactured foods (e.g. flour as a thickener or 'filler' in soups and sauces, and sometimes even in curry powder).

By law, wheat and its derivatives must be included in the ingredients label of any food manufactured to be sold in the EU. Derivatives of wheat include:

- all cereals of the *Triticum* species:
  - *Triticum spelta L* (spelt),
  - *Triticum polonicum L* (kamut),
- bran, wheat bran, wheat gluten, wheat germ,
- cereal filler, cereal binder, cereal protein,
- couscous,
- farina,
- flour, wholewheat flour, wheat flour, wheat starch,
- rusk,
- semolina, durum wheat semolina,

- starch, modified starch, hydrolysed starch, food starch, edible starch,
- vegetable protein, vegetable starch, vegetable gum*,
- wheat, durum wheat.

* Those labelled as guar gum or carageenan gum are wheat- and gluten-free.

WHEAT SUBSTITUTES

If you can tolerate rye, oats, barley, corn and rice, you can eat baked products, cereals and pastas using these grains in place of wheat. In addition, unusual grains and flours such as amaranth, arrowroot, bean, buckwheat, lentil, millet, pea, potato, quinoa and soya, as well as groundnuts and seeds (e.g. pumpkin and sunflower), may be used in interesting combinations to make baked products and cereals. Many of the commercial wheat-free products are based on these ingredients. Less common and rather more difficult to cook with are sago and tapioca flours. Banana flour and chestnut flour are also available.

Cakes and biscuits made without wheat are rarely as successful as those with wheat, because they do not rise as well and often have an inferior texture. In recent years, though, specialist food manufacturers have made considerable improvements to the substitute commercial mixes and preparations. Many of these companies will send free samples of their products on request.

Wheat is contained in manufactured and processed foods where it is used for its versatile properties as a processing aid, a binder or a filler or as a carrier for flavourings and spices. Examples of items where wheat *may* be a 'hidden' ingredient include:

artificial cream	ketchup	paté
baked beans	malt vinegar	potato waffles
canned meats	meat pies	processed cheese
curry powder	muesli	sausages
dry roasted nuts	mustards	Scotch eggs
fruit pie filling	packet soups	suet
haggis		

Malt is a by-product of barley or other grains; therefore products containing this should be avoided.

You will find that many of the special products that are manufactured for gluten-free diets are made from de-glutenised wheat. Remember that these are *not* suitable if you are on a wheat-free diet.

AVOIDING GLUTEN

Coeliac disease and the skin condition dermatitis herpetiformis are the two main conditions that require strict adherence to a gluten-free diet. To help its members (and others) steer clear of food products that contain gluten, Coeliac UK publishes *The Gluten-free Food & Drink Directory.* This is a small handbook (available in ordinary and in large print) containing a comprehensive list of manufactured products that are gluten-free. It is published annually and in between times there are regular updates about product changes. The handbook is available from Coeliac UK (contact details in Appendix 1).

Gluten-free foods on prescription

A range of gluten-free products, including breads, pastas, biscuits, pizza bases and cake mixes, are available on prescription at your GP's discretion. A full list of prescribable products can be obtained from your dietitian, from Coeliac UK or from most pharmacist/chemist shops.

Substitute foods

Gluten-free substitutes usually supply approximately the same amount of vitamins and minerals as the foods they replace. They are prepared with special care, following good manufacturing practice guidelines, to prevent contamination with ingredients that contain gluten. Quite a few of them are also formulated to be free from other ingredients that commonly cause allergic reactions in susceptible people, such as milk and egg. Later in this chapter is a list of types of wheat-free and gluten-free products that are available.

Top tips

- A full and regularly updated list of products available on prescription can be obtained from Coeliac UK.
- Don't forget to ask manufacturers and supermarkets for their 'free from' lists. There are probably many foods stocked in supermarkets that will be suitable for your special diet but are not marketed as such.

- Most pharmacist/chemist shops have a list of wheat- and gluten-free products available (some on prescription and some to buy over the counter or by mail order).
- Contact Coeliac UK if you require gluten-free communion wafers.
- Watch out for cross-contamination. It can easily occur with foods such as bread. The crumbs seem to get everywhere. For example, if you share your butter with people who eat ordinary bread, you can pick up bread crumbs left behind by their knives! Ensure that your foods are stored and prepared away from those containing wheat and gluten (see Chapter 15, 'Cross-contamination').

LABELLING

In the European Union, gluten-containing grains – including wheat – must, by law, be listed in the ingredients label. The legislation covers all pre-packaged manufactured foods but not those sold loose, such as bakery, butchery or delicatessen items. (See Chapter 9 for more about this.)

SPECIAL DIETARY PRODUCTS (wheat-free and gluten-free)

I have not included a specific listing of products made for wheat- and gluten-free diets as I did in the first edition of this book. The reason for this is that products tend to change, and many new ones regularly appear on the market, so by the time you read this edition it will not be fully up to date and you may miss out on new products that have become available.

It is more useful to know where to find out about the availability of products.

Many of the companies making wheat- and gluten-free products have an informative website, and offer newsletters, recipes and recipe cards, cookery demonstrations to attend or to watch on video or DVD, starter-pack samples on request and many other products, information and services.

Wheat- and/or gluten-free foods available include:

Baking and cooking

baking mix	breadcrumbs	pancake mix
baking powder	cake mix	pastry mix
bread mix	fruit loaf	scone mix

Sweet foods

biscuits, cookies, wafer bars,
    macaroons
cakes
Christmas puddings, cakes
    and mince pies

Danish pastries
fruit pies
ice-cream cones
jam tarts
steamed puddings

Savoury foods

bread – fresh, longlife, part-baked,
    sliced, unsliced
breadsticks
cheese straws
crackers
crispbreads
curry sauces
pasta

pies, quiches
pizza
ready-meals
sausage rolls
snack pots
speciality breads and bakery –
    baguettes, rolls, croissant
stuffings

Cereals

a selection of cereals

Snacks

cereal bars
pretzels

snack bars

This is just a selection of what's on offer. The availability, accessibility and taste of these products are improving all the time.

Getting your wheat- and gluten-free products

- Some are available on prescription at your GP's discretion. It may be worth getting a prepaid 'season ticket' certificate, depending on the quantity and frequency with which they are prescribed (see Chapter 17).
- Buy or order from your pharmacist or chemist.

Table 10.6 Companies making wheat- and gluten-free products

Manufacturer	Customer Careline	Website
Bakers Delight	01482 227439	www.bakers-delight.co.uk
Community Foods Ltd	020 8450 9419	www.communityfoods.co.uk
Doves Farm	01488 684880	www.dovesfarm.co.uk
General Dietary Ltd	020 8336 2323	www.ener-g.com
Gluten Free Foods Ltd	020 8953 4444	www.glutenfree-foods.co.uk
Heron Quality Foods Ltd	0116 867 4713	www.glutenfreedirect.com
Innovative Solutions	01260 222104	www.innovative-solutions.org.uk
Juvela (SHS)	0151 228 1992	www.juvela.co.uk
Karen's Cakes	020 8203 8049	—
Moilas UK	0845 0589850	www.moilas.co.uk
Novartis Medical Nutrition	01403 324134	www.biaglut.co.uk
Nutricia Dietary Care	01225 711801	www.glutafin.co.uk
Nutrition Point Ltd	07041 544044	www.nutritionpoint.co.uk
Orgran	—	www.orgran.com
Ultrapharm Ltd	01491 570 000	www.gfdiet.co.uk
Village Bakery of Melmerby	01768 889437	www.village-bakery.com and www.ok-foods.co.uk
Wellfoods of Barnsley Ltd	01226 381712	www.bake-it.com

It is worth noting that many products manufactured by these companies are also suitable for multiple-allergen-avoidance diets.

- Buy or order from your local healthfood store.
- Increasingly available from supermarkets – including own-brand products.
- From suppliers such as Goodness Direct (contact details in Appendix 1) through their website or from their catalogue by mail order or telephone.
- Direct from the manufacturers (listed in Table 10.6; available online, by mail order or telephone.

SOYA-FREE DIET

Soya (also referred to as soy) is a legume from the food family *Leguminosae* (see Chapter 12, 'Cross-reactivity and Food Families'). It is a rare cause of anaphylaxis in the UK but when it does occur, complete avoidance of soya and its derivatives is necessary. This can be restrictive because in recent years it has become a major component of manufactured foods.

Examples of manufactured foods that may contain soya include:

biscuits	Japanese food (contains miso)
bread and bakery items	paté
cakes	processed meats
Chinese food (contains soya sauce)	seasoned foods
cold delicatessen meats	teriyaki sauce

The ingredients to avoid are:

lecithin/soya lecithin (E322)	soya oil (especially cold-pressed)
miso	soya protein
soy/soya	soya protein isolate
soya albumin	soya sauce
soya bean sprouts	soya-based infant formula
soya beans	tempeh
soya flour	tofu
soya milk	vegetable protein, hydrolysed
soya nuts	vegetable protein, textured

If a manufactured, pre-packed product that is to be sold in the EU contains soya, this must, by law, be clearly listed on its ingredients label.

EATING OUT

If you are on a soya-free diet, eating out will probably be difficult unless dishes are made only from fresh ingredients. For ideas on how to eat out safely, see Chapters 14 ('Eating Away from Home') and 15 ('Cross-contamination').

TOILETRIES

Toiletries, perfumes and cosmetics containing soya or soya derivatives will be labelled according to the International Nomenclature of Cosmetic Ingredients (INCI). See Chapter 9 ('Food Labelling') for these names, which will enable you to identify them.

ALTERNATIVE FOODS

The following information should expand your diet, helping to make it more balanced. (If you are allergic to cow's milk as well as soya, this information will be particularly useful.)

Soya-free milks
Soya-free milks are generally based on oats, rice, coconut, peas, nuts, potato, chufa or quinoa.

Manufacturer	Product
Allergycare	*Rice* milk
Bart Spices	*Coconut* milk
Blue Dragon Foods	Tinned *coconut* milk, fat-reduced *coconut* milk
Clearspring	Imagine: Rice Dream *rice* milk: original, vanilla, chocolate, carob, calcium-enriched. Range includes 1 litre and lunchbox size: original, chocolate, vanilla
Evernat	Organic *almond* drink; organic *hazelnut* drink; organic *quinoa* drink
First Foods	*Oat* milk

Manufacturer	Product
Oatly	*Oat* drink: vanilla, chocolate
Plamil Foods	White Sun: *pea* protein alternative to milk: sweetened, unsweetened
Provamel	*Rice* drink with or without milk
Tiger White	*Chufa* milk: sweetened and unsweetened
Vance's Darifree	*Potato* milk powder: original, chocolate
Vitariz	Organic *rice* drink

Alternatively, try making your own nut milks. Recipes for other home-made milks can be found in any vegan cookbook. (See Appendix 3 for a list of recipe books.)

Soya-free spreads

There is a good range of soya-free and dairy-free spreads, including supermarket own-brand varieties. Remember to read the ingredients list if you have other food allergies.

Other soya-free foods

'Cheeses'

- Rice cheese slices, from Galaxy Foods. (Note, though, that they contain casein, which you should avoid if you are also allergic to cow's milk.)

Nutritional yeast-flakes

- Engevita Nutritional Flakes, from Marigold Healthfoods, are available from most healthfood shops. (See this chapter's section 'Dairy-free diet' for details.) These are useful as a 'cheese' flavouring.

Yoghurts and desserts

- Oat-based soya-free dairy-free 'ice-cream': Cornish ice-cream and choc ice on a stick (called Supreme), made by First Foods.

Cream

- Single cream – oat-based soya-free and dairy-free. made by First Foods.

ORAL ALLERGY SYNDROME

Oral allergy syndrome (OAS) is an allergic reaction to certain proteins in a variety of fruit, vegetables and nuts. Symptoms are usually confined to the lips, mouth, tongue and throat, and are usually treated successfully with antihistamines. A very small number of people may develop anaphylaxis, requiring urgent medical treatment including adrenaline.

Any food can cause OAS but it is usually fresh fruit and vegetables, especially if they are unpeeled. Foods are often safe to eat once they are cooked, as the proteins responsible for the reaction 'denature' (change their form) with heat.

Being allergic to pollens is also associated with certain fresh fruits and vegetables because they have similar protein structures. Your allergy specialist will help you to identify which pollens you are allergic to, which may help when trying to exclude the foods most commonly associated with a particular pollen allergy. You will need to exclude only foods that cause symptoms.

A common example of a person with OAS is someone who has a reaction when they eat any of the following: raw apples, apricots, cherries, kiwi, nectarines, pears, peaches, carrots, celery, fennel, parsley, peppers and almonds.

Foods most commonly associated with pollen allergy and oral allergy syndrome are listed in Table 10.7.

If you can eat a food without any problems, continue to do so, even if it appears in the lists in Table 10.7.

LATEX–FRUIT–POLLEN SYNDROME

People who are allergic to latex may experience allergic reactions to certain pollens and a variety of fresh fruits, vegetables and nuts. This is because the allergens are very similar. This is known as cross-reactivity (see Chapter 12).

Foods most commonly implicated include banana, kiwi, melons and papaya; avocado, carrot, celery, potato and tomato; chestnut and

Table 10.7 Foods commonly associated with pollen allergy and OAS

Birch pollen allergy	Ragweed pollen allergy
Apples, apricots, cherries, kiwi, nectarines, peaches, pears, plums, uncooked prunes; carrots, celery, coriander, fennel, parsley, parsnips, peppers, potatoes; almonds, hazelnuts and walnuts	Banana, cantaloupe and honeydew melon, watermelon; courgettes and cucumber Even dandelions or chamomile tea can cause a reaction because they belong to the same plant family. However, this allergy is found only in the USA
Alder pollen allergy	
Apples, cherries, peaches, pears; celery and parsley; almonds and hazelnuts	**Grass pollen allergy**
	Melon (all types), oranges; tomatoes
	Mugwort pollen allergy
	Carrots, celery, coriander, fennel, parsley, peppers and sunflower

hazelnut. Reactions can range from mild to anaphylaxis; they require a formal diagnosis so that the most appropriate rescue medication can be prescribed.

KIWI ALLERGY

There is research as well as reports of reactions indicating that kiwi fruit seems to be a significant food allergen – not only in its link with latex but also as an allergen in its own right. Take care when eating foods you have not prepared yourself, as there is a significant risk of cross-contamination. Kiwi is used in starters, fruit salads, sweet sauces, jams and jellies. Its presence could easily be hidden, and it can be legally undeclared in a manufactured food if it is part of an ingredient within that product. For example, if kiwi was used in a fruit jelly and that fruit jelly was less than 2% of the finished product, legally the label only has to say 'fruit jelly' and the kiwi will not be listed specifically. As with all non-packaged foods such as delicatessen, butchery and bakery items, the law does not require the ingredients to be listed (see Chapter 9).

CELERY ALLERGY

Celery is one of the most common foods to cause OAS in adults in mainland Europe. Allergy to celeriac (the root) is more common than to celery (the stalk) but both can cause severe reactions. All sources of celery should be avoided, including that in soups and stock cubes and when used as celery salt or in powder form.

Manufactured foods must tell you on the label if they contain celery but foods not packaged, such as bakery, butchery or delicatessen items, will not carry an ingredients list so should be avoided. When eating food you have not prepared yourself, do so with extreme caution because celery may be used in soups, stock, sauces, marinades, casseroles, stews and many other dishes. You should also consider cross-contamination issues (see Chapter 15).

MUSTARD ALLERGY

Mustard allergy, which is quite rare in the UK, is more common in mainland Europe where mustard is used more. If you react to mustard, you should avoid it in all its forms: mustard, mustard powder, mustard leaves and seeds, mustard oil and foods containing any of these. Manufactured foods have to tell you on the label if they contain mustard but any foods not packaged – such as bakery, butchery or delicatessen items – will not carry an ingredients list so should be avoided. When eating food you have not prepared yourself, do so with extreme caution because mustard is often used in soups, stock, sauces, marinades and in many recipes. You should also consider cross-contamination issues (see Chapter 15).

SULPHITES

Sulphur dioxide (E220) and other sulphites (E221, E222, E223, E224, E226, E227 and E228) are used in a wide range of manufactured foods, including soft drinks, cordials and squashes, sausages, burgers, and dried fruit and vegetables. They are also added to beer and to grape juice for wine.

Since November 2005 food labelling laws require pre-packaged foods sold in the EU to show clearly on the label if a product contains sulphur dioxide or sulphites at levels above 10mg per kilogram or per litre.

Anaphylaxis caused by sulphites is unlikely, and adverse reactions have been linked mainly to asthma. Nevertheless, they are included in this book because sulphites are one of the top 12 (soon to be 14) allergens in the EU (see Chapter 9).

MULTIPLE FOOD ALLERGIES

A significant proportion of people who have a food allergy have more than one allergy; and some have many food allergies. This can be extremely difficult to manage and the impact on their life is great. Their diet can become nutritionally deficient and their food not very tasty.

If you are one of these people, it is more important than ever that you see a dietitian, who will be able to provide tailored advice and information regarding:

- nutrition
- replacement foods
- recipes
- meal plans
- reading food labels
- shopping and cooking

(See also Chapter 8.)

11
Allergy Prevention
Pregnancy, breast-feeding, formula milks and weaning

If you are planning an addition to your family, you will probably want to know how likely it is that the new baby might develop an allergy of some sort. You can then consider aspects of nutrition before conception, during pregnancy, during breast-feeding and when weaning the baby.

ATOPY

'Atopy' is the term for an inherited tendency that makes it more likely that a person will develop an allergy. Not everyone who has atopy is necessarily going to develop an allergy but they are more likely to do so than someone without that tendency. Common allergic disorders include asthma, eczema, hay-fever, perennial rhinitis (like hay-fever but it lasts all year) and food alleregy. The potential for an infant inheriting an atopic condition is estimated as:

    10–15% if neither parent is atopic
    30–50% if one parent is atopic
    60–80% if both parents are atopic

A number of family studies have found that the mother's atopy is more likely than the father's to affect the next generation. This may be because the fetus is exposed to an allergic environment while in the womb.

THE FATHER'S DIET

If you are planning for a baby with your partner, it is important to eat a varied balanced diet that fulfils all nutritional needs, for at least three months before conception. This is important for optimum healthy sperm production.

ADVICE FOR THE MOTHER

Pre-conception and pregnancy

If you are trying for a baby it is essential that you have a healthy, balanced diet. You should also take folic acid supplements as recommended by the Department of Health. Your dietitian, midwife, practice nurse or GP can advise you about this.

If you or your partner or siblings of the baby-to-be are atopic (have eczema, asthma, hay-fever or food allergy), the Department of Health recommends that you avoid peanuts during your pregnancy.

At present this is the only advice we have about avoiding certain foods during pregnancy for an allergy-preventative effect. Remember, though, that some other foods should be avoided during pregnancy for other health reasons – for example, paté and soft cheeses.

Women who cut some foods out of their diet while pregnant – hoping to reduce the risk of the baby developing allergies – have a higher risk of premature and low-birth-weight babies. So do not restrict your diet unless you have been advised otherwise by your doctor and have adequate supervision from a dietitian.

Breast or bottle?

Breast-feeding is recommended as the first choice of infant nutrition from birth by the World Health Organization (WHO) and by various European and UK medical advisory bodies. There are many advantages to breast-feeding, and there is some evidence to suggest that it may also have an allergy-preventative effect.

Exclusive breast-feeding for six months (a minimum of four months – 17 weeks) is recommended. By 'exclusive breast-feeding' we mean breast-feeding alone, so no formula feeding and no weaning in the first six months. Despite this recommendation, however, we know that in practice many babies are not breast-fed, or only partially breast-fed, so what should those babies be having?

Bottle-feeding There is evidence that babies from atopic families who are bottle-fed should have a hydrolysed formula or partially hydrolysed formula. This is because there is evidence that these milks reduce the risk of allergic disease developing. There are, however, no UK Department of Health guidelines about this as yet; the guidelines we do have are European and/or from the World Health Organization.

Because of this, prescribing these hydrolysed formulas for the prevention of allergy will be at your doctor's discretion. They can be purchased from a chemist but for many the cost may be prohibitive.

Your paediatric dietitian will be able to advise you about the most appropriate infant formula milk for your baby.

FORMULA MILKS FOR THE ALLERGIC INFANT

Infant formulas

Infant formulas are designed specifically to meet the nutritional needs of a growing infant. They comply fully with the UK regulations for infant formulas and are suitable for use as the sole source of nourishment for a young infant or as part of a mixed diet given to older infants and young children. A dietitian can help you make the correct choice of formula for your infant if you are in doubt.

The UK manufacturers of all infant products, including baby formulas, have removed nut and peanut derivatives from them to reduce the risk of early allergic sensitisation.

Soya protein formulas

Soya formulas are no longer recommended as the first choice for the prevention (or treatment) of cow's milk allergy.

In January 2004 England's Chief Medical Officer advised that, owing to the natural phytoestrogens (oestrogen-like substances) present in soya, soya-based formulas should not be given to infants under 6 months. The exceptions to this include vegan infants and infants refusing, or unable to tolerate, other formulas that would usually have been prescribed.

The associated risks of phytoestrogens are related to the quantity of soya consumed per weight of the infant. Therefore, as the child grows and the amount of formula reduces with the introduction of a mixed diet, so the possible risks reduce.

Another issue with soya is that some infants who have a milk allergy will also be allergic to soya milks.

Dental implications of soya infant formulas

Because soya infant formulas contain glucose syrups rather than lactose (which is the sugar occurring naturally in cow's milk), they are thought to have a greater potential to contribute to tooth decay (dental caries). It has been suggested that the soya formula should be given as drink, not as a comforter, if the development of dental caries is to be reduced. The longer the contact of the soya formula with the teeth, the greater the risk of tooth decay, so the baby's teeth should be brushed after each and every feed.

Protein hydrolysate formulas

These are specifically designed for babies with an intolerance or allergy to milk. They often contain cow's milk in which the proteins have been broken down by the process called hydrolysis, which makes them far less allergenic. (They can be extensively or partially hydrolysed.) These formulas are *not* suitable for infants who are known to have a severe allergy to cow's milk.

Amino acid formulas

Infants who cannot tolerate a protein hydrolysate can be given a formula made up of amino acids (the building blocks from which proteins are made). Amino acid formulas are sometimes called 'elemental formulas'. Because cow's milk is not used, this type of formula should not trigger an allergy.

Alternatives to cow's milk

It is essential to use a formula designed for infants. Soya milk, rice milk, oat milk, goat's milk and sheep's milk that are often used by older children and adults who are unable to tolerate, or choose not to take, cow's milk are not suitable for an infant because they do not contain adequate nutrition.

Goat's milk formula

In general, an infant who is allergic to cow's milk will often develop an allergy to goat's milk if this is used as a substitute – this is because the proteins are very similar. Therefore, goat's milk formula is not usually recommended as an alternative to cow's milk or cow's milk formula. Since March 2007 it has been banned from sale in the UK.

IF COW'S MILK FORMULA IS UNSUITABLE

Although this chapter is about the *prevention* of allergy, I have included information on which formula milks are suitable for the treatment/management of cow's milk allergy and intolerance. This is to reduce the confusion that exists about all the different formula

Hydrolysed formula

For allergy prevention

Recommended by the World Health Organization and European agencies for high-risk infants where the mother, father or siblings have documented allergic disease – eczema, asthma, hay-fever (rhinitis), food allergy

Extensively hydrolysed formula

Casein hydrolysates:

- Prejestimil [Mead Johnson]
- Nutramigen [Mead Johnson]
- Nutramigen stage 2 (over 6 months) [Mead Johnson]

Partially hydrolysed formula

- NAN H.A. 1 (0–6 months) [Nestle]
- NAN H.A. 2 (over 6 months)

For the treatment of cow's milk protein allergy and intolerance

Extensively hydrolysed formula

Casein hydrolysates:

- Prejestimil [Mead Johnson]
- Nutramigen [Mead Johnson]
- Nutramigen stage 2 (over 6 months) [Mead Johnson]

Whey hydrolysates:

- Pepti [Cow & Gate]
- Pepti-Junior [Cow & Gate]

The whey-based hydrolysates are not hydrolysed as extensively as the casein-based ones. Because of this, they may be accepted more readily by infants where the taste is an issue.

The most appropriate hydrolysed formula will depend on the degree of hydrolysis and the fat and lactose content required.

Soya formula

- Farleys Soya Formula [Heinz]
- Infasoy [Cow & Gate]
- Isomil [Abbott]
- Prosobee [Mead Johnson]
- Wysoy [SMA]

Infants 0–6 months

Soya formula should not be prescribed except in exceptional circumstances. For example, infants:

- of vegan parents who are not breast-feeding
- who are refusing all other formulas that would otherwise be tolerated

Infants 6–12 months

Soya formula can be given if the infant is:

- refusing other formula milks
- severely allergic to cow's milk

From 6 months of age other soya products such as soya yoghurts, cheeses and puddings can be given as part of the infant's diet if soya is tolerated.

Infants over 12 months

- Soya formula can be given freely.
- Soya products can be taken as part of the diet.

Elemental formula

An 'elemental' formula is made up of protein, fat and carbohydrates in their simplest forms, with the addition of vitamins, minerals and trace elements. It is used for the management of severe milk allergy where there is a risk of a severe reaction to the cow's milk protein in the formula.

- Neocate (0–12 months) [SHS]
- Neocate Advance (1–12 years) [SHS]

Low-lactose formula

Low-lactose formula is prescribed for infants who cannot tolerate the milk sugar, lactose.

- Pepti [Cow & Gate]
- Enfamil Lactofree [Mead Johnson]
- Galactomin 17 [SHS]
- SMA LF [SMA]

milks available and their uses. However, for detailed information, contact the manufacturers of the formula.

Peanut allergy

The Committee on Toxicity of Chemicals in Food, Consumer Products and the Environment (COT) was commissioned to look into the consumption of peanuts and peanut products by pregnant and breast-feeding women, infants and young children. They looked particularly at early exposure to peanut products and the risk of developing peanut allergy later in life. In June 1998 they reported the following:

- Atopy is an important factor in the development of peanut allergy.
- There is insufficient evidence available to give definite advice about not eating peanuts during pregnancy and breast-feeding or in early childhood.
- Advice, which is precautionary, recommends that:
  - women with allergic disease, or those with an allergic partner or child, may wish to avoid eating peanuts and peanut products during pregnancy and breast-feeding,
  - in common with the advice for all children, a susceptible baby should be breast-fed exclusively for the first four to six months,
  - during weaning, and until they are at least three years of age, infants should not be exposed to peanuts or peanut products.

Refined peanut oils should not contain peanut allergens. The use of products containing these oils in food, ointments or creams should not therefore result in an allergic reaction. In the extremely rare event of a reaction, it is most likely that it would be mild. If you are still worried, though, seek advice from your NHS allergy clinic or specialist for specific individual advice. (See also 'Peanut-free and nut-free diets' in Chapter 10.)

WEANING

It is recommended that weaning should not start before four months (17 weeks) and preferably not until six months.

It is also recommended that low-allergenic weaning foods should be given before the foods more frequently associated with food allergy, particularly if weaning is begun before the baby is six months old. They include:

- apricot
- banana
- carrot
- chicken
- lamb
- melon
- peach
- pear
- potato
- rice
- swede
- sweet potato
- turkey
- other meats and vegetables

The following foods are more often associated with allergy, so should be introduced only after the first foods have been given. Note that peanuts should be avoided *completely* in atopic infants until they are three years of age.

- celery
- cereals containing gluten (wheat, rye, barley, oats, spelt, kamut or their hybridised strains)
- cow's milk
- crustaceans
- egg
- fish
- mustard
- nuts (almonds, walnut, cashew, pecan, Brazil, pistachio, macadamia, Queensland nut)
- peanuts
- sesame
- soya

The following is the summary of the consensus statement from the Food Allergy and Intolerance Special Group of the British Dietetic Association, and should be used as a guide. Discuss it with your dietitian, who will be able to offer you individually tailored advice for your infant.

PRACTICAL DIETARY PREVENTION STRATEGIES FOR INFANTS AT RISK OF DEVELOPING ALLERGIC DISEASES

Summary

The nutritional advice below is for infants who do not already have suspected or proven food allergy or allergic disease, but who are at risk of developing food allergy because of parental or sibling atopy.

- Mothers should eat a healthy, balanced diet during pregnancy and breast-feeding, including all major allergens, although those whose babies are at highest risk may wish to avoid peanuts

- Ideally, breast-feeding should be the sole source of nutrition until the baby is 6 months old

- Recommended alternatives to breast milk are partially or extensively hydrolysed formula milks; infants at highest risk should be given extensively hydrolysed casein formula milk

- Other milks, including soya, goat's or standard cow's milk formulas, or non-formula off-the-shelf cow's, goat's, sheep, soya or rice milk, must not be given

- Weaning should never commence before the age of 17 weeks. Any solids introduced between 4 and 6 months should be the traditional low-allergenic weaning foods

- From the age of 6 months, once weaning has become established with low-allergenic foods, the introduction of high-allergenic foods into the diet can begin

- High-allergenic foods such as wheat, egg and milk should be commenced by adding in each food singly, starting with a small amount and introducing no more than one new allergenic food at a time

- At all times, experts' guidelines on the introduction of different textures into the diet must be followed in order to ensure that the child develops appropriate chewing and swallowing techniques associated with eating solid food

- Infants being introduced to solids from the age of 6 months should commence with low-allergenic weaning foods but rapidly progress in order to meet 'texture milestones' and not further delay the introduction of high-allergenic foods

- By the age of 12 months all the major allergenic foods, which would normally be suitable for a child of this age, should have been introduced (with the exception of peanuts)

- There is no evidence that delaying the introduction of high-allergenic foods beyond the age of 6 months is beneficial to at-risk infants
- Delaying weaning beyond 6 months could adversely affect the normal dietary and developmental milestones essential to establishing a good varied diet
- **Infants with a suspected or proven food allergy, or other allergic disease, will need individual assessment and advice and are not covered by these guidelines**

Reproduced, with minor amendments, from the summary consensus statement by the Food Allergy and Intolerance Special Group of the British Dietetic Association

As you can see from the information included in this chapter, we still have a lot to learn about preventing allergies in infants. It is an area where much research is currently underway and hopefully one day we will have a better understanding of it and be able to give more firm advice.

In the meantime, always seek advice from your specialist for the most appropriate infomation and guidance for your baby.

12
Cross-reactivity and Food Families

Cross-reactivity is a condition in which the body mistakes one substance for another of similar or identical chemical composition. Allergens that cross-react with one another always have a common chemical structure or group. These allergens may be from the same food family (genetically related) or from a different food family (not genetically related).

This chapter is included in the book so that, if you are having reactions to which a dietary cause has not been found, the information may give you a starting point for investigations. Do not cut foods out of your diet without any evidence that it is those foods that may be causing reactions. And always discuss your thoughts first with the doctor at your allergy clinic. Keeping food and symptom diaries, having skin-prick and blood tests and food challenge tests are all ways of investigating, diagnosing and confirming food allergies.

COMMON CROSS-REACTIONS BETWEEN FOODS IN THE SAME GROUP

If you are allergic to one item in a food family listed below, it is likely you will be allergic to all members of that family, and should therefore avoid them. Note that this is not the rule for other food families – only these four:

- crustaceans
- fish
- animal milks
- eggs

If you are allergic to fish, you should avoid fish eggs. (But you may eat birds' eggs.) Remember that eggs are *not* dairy foods.

COMMON CROSS-REACTIONS BETWEEN FOODS IN DIFFERENT GROUPS

Sometimes foods can cross-react across food families because they contain proteins of very similar or identical structure. If foods are found to cross-react, they should be avoided. If they are tolerated, you can usually continue to eat them. The exception to this is peanuts and nuts: if you have an allergy to a peanut or nut, *all* peanuts and nuts should be avoided. The three food groups in which cross-reactivity can occur are:

- peanuts and other nuts;
- banana, chestnut, kiwi, melons, papaya; avocado, carrot, celery, potato, tomato,; hazelnut (and latex and various pollens; see the section 'Latex–fruit–pollen syndrome' in Chapter 10);
- certain fruit, vegetables and nuts (see the section 'Oral allergy syndrome' in Chapter 10).

Food families – botanical and animal – are listed in Table 12.1 for your information only. They may provide a clue if you are having reactions to a food and cannot work out what is causing the reaction. The answer may lie in the food families listed, but then again it may not. Your dietitian will be able to help you interpret these food families if you want more information.

Table 12.1 List of food families

Botanical food families

Actinidiaceae	Kiwi
Banana (Musae)	Banana, plantain
Birch (Betulaceae)	Hazelnut
Boraginaceae	Borage
Brazil nut (Lecythidaceae)	Brazil nut
Buckwheat (Polygonaceae)	Buckwheat, rhubarb, sorrel
Cactus (Cactaceae) .	Fig, prickly pear
Cashew (Anacardiaceae)	Cashew, mango, pistachio
Citrus (Rutacea)	Angostura, clementine, citron, grapefruit, kumquat, lemon, lime, orange, tangerine, ugli fruit

Table 12.1 List of food families (*continued*)

Composite Family (Compositae)	Artichoke, calendula peta, chamomile, chicory, endive, escarole, lettuce, salsify, sesame seeds, sunflower seeds
Flax (Linaceae)	Flaxseed
Fungi	Baker's yeast, brewer's yeast, mushrooms
Ginger (Zingiberaceae)	Arrowroot, cardamom, ginger, turmeric
Gooseberry (Grossulariaceae)	Blackcurrant, gooseberry, redcurrant
Goosefoot (Chenopodiaceae)	Quinoa, spinach, sugar beet
Gourd (Cucurbitaceae)	Cantaloupe, cucumber, honeydew melon, pawpaw, papaya, pumpkin, squash, watermelon
Grains, grasses, cereals	Bamboo shoots, barley (barley malt), cane sugar, chestnut, corn, lemon grass, ling nut, millet, oats, rice, rye, sorghum, tapioca, water chestnut, wheat
Grape (Vitaceae)	Brandy, champagne, cognac, crème of tartar, grape (currants, grape leaf, raisins, sultanas), wine, wine vinegar
Heather (Ericaceae)	Blueberry, cranberry
Honeysuckle (Caprifoliaceae)	Elderberry
Iris (Iridaceae)	Saffron
Laurel (Lauraceae)	Avocado, bay leaves, cinnamon
Legumes (Leguminosae)	Adzuki bean, alfalfa, alfalfa bean sprouts, black-eyed pea, black turtle beans, carob, fava beans, fenugreek, field pea, garbanzo bean (chickpea), great northern bean, green bean, green pea, guar gum, jicama, kidney bean, lentil, liquorice, lima bean, lupin, mung bean (mungo beans, mung bean sprouts), navy bean, peanut, pinto bean, soybean, split pea, string bean, tamarind
Lily (Liliaceae)	Asparagus, chives, garlic, leek, onion, shallot

Table 12.1 List of food families (*continued*)

Mint (Labiatae)	Apple mint, lavender, marjoram, oregano, rosemary, sage, thyme
Morning glory (Convolvulaceae)	Sweet potato, yam
Mulberry (Artocapaceae)	Breadfruit, fig, mulberry
Mustard (Cruciferae)	Broccoli, Brussels sprout, cabbage, cauliflower, Chinese cabbage, horseradish, kale, mustard, radish, turnip, watercress
Myrtle (Myrtaceae)	Allspice, cloves, guava, paprika, pimento
Nightshade (Solanaceae)	Anaheim pepper, aubergine, banana pepper, bell pepper, brinjal, cayenne, chili pepper, green pepper, ground cherry, habanera pepper, hatch pepper, jalapeno pepper, paprika, pimento, potato (all varieties except sweet potato), red pepper, sweet pepper, tabasco, tomato
Nutmeg (Myristicaceae)	Mace, nutmeg
Olive (Oleaceae)	Olive
Orchid (Orchidaceae)	Vanilla
Palm (Palmaceae)	Coconut, palm
Parsley (Apiceae)	Angelica, anise, caraway, carrots, celeriac, celery, celery seed, chervil, coriander, cumin, dill, fennel, parsley, parsnips, water celery
Pepper (Piperaceae)	Black pepper, pink peppercorn, white pepper
Pine (Pinaceae and Coniferae)	Juniper berry, pine nut, pinion nut
Pineapple (Bromeliaceae)	Pineapple
Poppy (Papaveraceae)	Poppy seed

Table 12.1 List of food families (*continued*)

Rose (Rosaceae)	Almond, apple, apricot, blackberry, boysenberry, cherry, dewberry, loganberry, nectarine, peach, pear, plum, prune, quince, raspberry, strawberry
Rubiaceae	Coffee
Stercula	Cocoa, cola bean
Walnut (Juglandaceae)	Butternut, hickory nut, pecan, walnut

Animal food families

Amphibia	Frog
Crustaceans	Crab, crawfish, crayfish, lobster, prawn, shrimp
Fowl	Chicken, duck, emu, grouse, guineafowl, ostrich, partridge, pea fowl, pheasant, pigeon, prairie chicken, quail, snipe, turkey, woodcock Eggs are included in this category
Fresh water fish	Big mouth bass, catfish, croaker, mullet, perch, pike, salmon, sun fish, trout, walleye, whitefish
Mammal	Bear, beef (veal, cow's milk, cheese and butter), buffalo (bison), caribou, deer (venison), elk, goat (goat's cheese, goat's milk), horse (mare's milk), lamb (mutton, ewe's milk and cheese), moose, opossum, pork (ham, bacon), rabbit (hare), raccoon, seal, squirrel
Mollusc	Abalone, clam, conch, mussel, oyster, periwinkle, quahog, scallop, snail, squid
Salt water fish	Amberjack, anchovy, blue fish, cod, drum, flounder, grouper, hake, halibut, herring, mackerel, mahi mahi, mullet, orange roughy, pompano, salmon, salt water trout, sardine, sheephead, snapper, striped bass, swordfish, tuna, whiting

13
Eating In

You could be forgiven for thinking that eating at home on a restricted diet is bland, boring and unimaginative. This is probably because it is all too easy to focus on the foods that you must avoid rather than those that are safe for you to eat. Unfortunately, the foods that you *can* eat never seem quite as appealing as those that you *can't*!

The information in this chapter will enable you to increase your food choices and add variety to your diet. Instead of feeling the odd one out at mealtimes, you will be able to share food and enjoy eating with your family.

HOW CAN I MAKE MY DIET MORE APPETISING?

Making food appetising both to you and to those you are catering for simply means cooking nutritious food that tastes and looks good. Although some recipes will need adapting by replacing certain ingredients with suitable alternatives, there will be many recipes that you can continue to use without making any changes. Experiment with new foods and special dietary products that are available, such as egg replacers or gluten-free items. And you can try out some new recipes, too.

Whether you want to prepare a snack, a gourmet dinner party or a birthday cake that everyone can eat, there are endless possibilities. There is plenty of scope for the reluctant cook, for those who love cooking and for those with a hectic lifestyle and no time to spend in the kitchen. You can continue to make use of fresh, dried, tinned, frozen and many convenience foods if you so desire.

Finding suitable foods and learning to make the most of what you can still eat are the key to an interesting and varied diet. It is easier than ever to achieve this now – many supermarkets now stock an increasing selection of 'special diet' foods, and healthfood shops and their range of products are becoming more abundant.

With the introduction of allergen-labelling legislation in 2005, it is now possible to eat foods that were once avoided because they might have contained undeclared ingredients. (Food labelling is discussed in Chapter 9.)

Supermarket 'free from' lists

Most supermarkets produce 'free from' lists. These are lists of all their own-brand foods that are free from a particular ingredient. 'Free from' lists are available free of charge and are updated regularly. (See Appendix 1 for contact details of the major supermarkets that provide this service.)

Always double-check the ingredients label on the product to ensure that it is still suitable for your particular diet. Ingredients sometimes change after the 'free from' list has been prepared – look out for 'New' or 'Improved' on the packaging. (See Chapter 9 for more information.)

Manufacturers' 'free from' lists

Many food manufacturers now produce their own 'free from' lists. This means that you can contact many of them direct to obtain a list of their products that are suitable for your particular diet. The manufacturers' contact details can be found on the packaging. It is usual for this to include the address, telephone number and website.

Specialist food companies

Many specialised food companies produce foods and ingredients that can be used as alternatives to those you have to avoid on a restricted diet. (Appendix 1 lists many of these companies.) You will be amazed at the choice.

This area of the food industry has been expanding rapidly in recent years and is still gaining momentum. If you can spend some time finding out about and keeping up to date with 'special diet' products, your dietary horizons will blossom. Contact Goodness Direct or log on to their website for a comprehensive product guide.

WHERE TO FIND OUT ABOUT 'SPECIAL DIET' PRODUCTS

- Goodness Direct.
- Chapter 10 and Appendix 1.
- Your dietitian.
- Your local allergy support group:
  - through the information and newsletters it provides,
  - by meeting and chatting with others who follow a special diet.

- Your local healthfood shop.
- By contacting and/or joining an association dedicated to food allergy (see Appendix 1).
- Your library.
- The Internet – there are various websites (see Appendix 2) that hold up-to-date information. (If you do not have access to the Internet, go to your local library who will either help you or be able to direct you to somewhere that can.)
- Your local pharmacist/chemist shop (choose a quiet time of day!).
- Your supermarket – take time to look thoroughly at what is available on the supermarket shelves, then discuss other possibilities with the manager.
- Health shows and fairs.

FINDING SUITABLE REPLACEMENT FOODS

Initially it will be trial and error to find replacement foods and ingredients that you like or are prepared to use. Some products may be unacceptable to you because of their taste, texture, price or availability. You may also have to cope with ingredients whose cooking properties are different from the products that they are replacing. Whatever the reason, do persevere. And keep trying new products developed for your particular allergy. For example, manufacturers of gluten-free products are constantly striving to produce gluten-free bread that tastes like the 'real thing' as well as expanding their range of other foods.

What about the cost?

Some companies will send you free samples of their products if you ask them, which is a good, cheap way to experiment with potential replacement foods. In some cases, they will keep your address on file and send you samples of new products they develop.

There are some state benefits and free prescriptions available for certain medical conditions, which can help with the cost of specialised products. This subject is discussed in Chapter 17.

What about my favourite recipes?

You can often continue to use your present recipes, replacing some ingredients as necessary. Be aware, though, that some recipes will need adapting. Some of these adapted recipes will be just the same or even an improvement on the original, while others will be a downright disaster. You just have to put this down to experience!

You can of course get cookery books specifically designed for special diets (see Appendix 3). They usually include a chapter on replacement ingredients. A bookshop will usually get these for you, or you can order them direct on the Internet if you prefer. Or your dietitian or allergy support group may well have some recipe books.

Manufacturers of specialised food products usually provide a recipe book on request. All the recipes have been tried and tested, which is particularly useful for the novice.

Cookery courses

Try to go on a cookery course. For wheat- and gluten-free cookery, contact Coeliac UK for details. For egg- and milk-free cookery – including cooking with dairy- and egg-free alternatives – contact the Vegan Society. Such courses will help you to learn how to cook within your dietary restrictions. (Contact details of these two organisations are in Appendix 1.)

Remember!

- If you are working in the same area that has been used to prepare foods to which you are allergic, or using the same utensils, they must be thoroughly cleaned to prevent cross-contamination (see Chapter 15).
- Plan meals enough in advance that you have all the required ingredients to make your chosen dish. This is especially important if some of the ingredients are not widely available.
- Eating in successfully is really down to how much preparatory work you do and how you use the information you have about your particular allergy or allergies. Start with one or two simple dishes and before long your very own special recipes will have reached gourmet heights and those eating with you will look forward to trying your latest creation. Like anything new, adapting to your new diet will take time but, with perseverance, it will become routine.
- The 'Eating In checklist' on the facing page will help you remember the important points in the early days, and you might find it useful to look at it again from time to time.

- Take photographs of your creations, write the recipe on the back and start your own cookbook, which you can lend to family, friends and carers.

By the time you have ticked all the boxes and spent a little time experimenting with recipes, your diet will no longer seem bland and unimaginative, and you will look forward with enthusiasm to the next innovation in your expanding recipe book.

MY EATING IN CHECKLIST

☐ I have seen a dietitian.

☐ I understand food labelling.

☐ I have a 'free from' list from all my local supermarkets and know how to use them.

☐ I have contacted food manufacturers for their 'free from' lists.

☐ I always double-check food labels when using 'free from' lists.

☐ I have obtained samples of replacement ingredients for special food products where they are available.

☐ I have tried replacement ingredients and foods.

☐ I have tried out lots of new recipes.

☐ I have joined an allergy support group.

☐ I have joined appropriate support organisations and receive regular newsletters from them.

☐ I have visited the library, bookshop or Internet websites for more information.

☐ I have checked with my GP or dietitian for information on any foods available on prescription for my allergy.

☐ I plan meals well in advance, especially if I know that I am going to be busy or if I am cooking for others.

☐ I always clean utensils and work-surfaces before I start preparing food.

☐ I have tried more than one type of replacement food rather than giving up on replacement foods because I didn't like the first couple that I tried.

14
Eating Away from Home

When you are on a restricted diet, eating away from home can be difficult. This may be due to the practicalities involved or because of other people's attitudes, ignorance and misunderstandings.

There is usually a way round most difficulties but it can sometimes be tedious and take away the pleasure of eating out. This chapter will help you to deal with issues that may occur in everyday situations so that you will be able to eat away from home safely and confidently.

'Eating out' encompasses many different settings, including the following:

- barbecue
- bed and breakfast
- Brownies/Cubs/Scouts
- buffet
- church
- cinema
- conference
- course
- dance
- dinner party
- fair or fête
- health club
- hospital
- hotel
- nursery
- party
- picnic
- pub
- restaurant
- sandwich bar
- school or school outing
- shopping trip
- take-away
- theatre
- tourist attractions
- travel
- university or college
- wedding

You will have to make specific arrangements that will vary according to where you are going and what you are doing, but below are some basic guidelines that you should always follow if the experience is to be as hassle-free and as safe as possible.

BASIC GUIDELINES FOR EATING OUT

- Understand your food allergy, and be able to answer questions about it competently and clearly when asked by those preparing food for you.
- Always contact, in advance, the person who is catering for you to tell them about your special diet. Clear written guidelines are ideal for minimising the risk of ambiguity and they can be kept for future reference. The person doing the catering – whether a friend, a colleague or a professional caterer – will then know that they are well prepared and be confident that the food they are providing is suitable.
- Try to persuade the caterer that making food for all members of the party in accordance with your diet will probably make life a lot easier for them as well as safer for you.
- Find out answers to questions you are unsure of before eating anything you may be allergic to.
- Do *not* under any circumstances eat any food prepared by someone else *unless you are sure* it is definitely safe for you.
- Check the ingredients of any manufactured foods used by the chef to ensure that they are all suitable.
- Have the confidence to say what is required to ensure that the food you consume is safe for you. If the caterer is unable or unwilling to provide what you need, suggest that you bring your own.
- Take your own food if it has been agreed with the person who usually does the catering. You can make this less conspicuous by:
  - making sure the person doing the catering and arranging the event knows in advance that you are doing this,
  - ensuring that your food looks the same as everyone else's by finding out in advance what the others will be eating and obtaining (e.g. borrowing from a restaurant) similar crockery so that yours doesn't look out of place,
  - taking your food earlier in the day to wherever you will be eating (cover it to prevent cross-contamination) and explain any issues both verbally and in writing to save time and trouble later when staff are often busy and perhaps less receptive,
  - or taking your food to the kitchen when you arrive at the function so that it can be served to you at the same time as

the rest of your party. (Make sure that those serving are
aware of the cross-contamination issues (see Chapter 15).)

- Don't avoid situations because they will involve eating; instead,
  plan well ahead so that food no longer becomes an issue.
- Speak to the chef direct rather than via the waiting staff, who
  will not necessarily relay your needs to the chef correctly.
- Take your own special ingredients, pans and utensils for the
  chef to use and any seasoning that will enhance the enjoyment
  of your food. (But give them plenty of notice!)
- Patronise the same restaurant/pub/eating house again if you
  have had a successful eating experience. It is better to return on
  a quieter day at a quieter time of day if possible (8 p.m. on a
  Saturday night with no forewarning is not a good time to ask
  for a special meal!).
- Be aware that food allergens can appear in the most unusual
  ways – so check:
  - communion wafers (they usually contain gluten),
  - home-made jams (they often contain butter – used to clarify
    the 'scum' during making),
  - mulled wine and cocktails (they could contain anything, and
    the fruit might have been cut on a board with allergens on it),
  - the sugar bowl (this almost certainly contains globules of
    milk).

If you are at risk of having an anaphylactic reaction:

- DO *carry your adrenaline at all times.*
- DO understand when and how to use adrenaline and be
  prepared to use it. (See Chapter 5, 'Your Anaphylaxis
  Contingency Plan'.)

Taking your own food

Remember that many establishments *will* allow you to take food that
you have prepared yourself, and they will heat it up for you if
required. If the food is covered in cling film, you can be sure it will be
completely safe, which means you can concentrate on enjoying yourself instead of worrying and the staff can relax!

SPECIAL OCCASIONS

If you are organising an important function such as a wedding, christening or anniversary, you will probably want to employ a caterer to prepare the food. Some caterers can be unhelpful or ignorant about food allergy but do not give up! There *are* caterers out there who are experienced in this aspect of food preparation and will be willing to cater for your special function. It is wise to plan the catering well ahead so that you have plenty of time to find someone you are happy with and trust to do exactly as you request. I am living proof of this: at my own wedding I had a completely dairy-free spread of delicious food.

GOING INTO HOSPITAL

You may, at some time in your life, have to go into hospital. This may be for a planned operation or it might be unexpected.

Whatever the case, you need to be aware that even hospitals are not always as informed as they should be about food allergies, cross-contamination issues and hidden allergens in foods. In some cases it may be necessary to take your own food with you, or get someone who usually caters for you to bring your food in each day.

SEVERE FOOD ALLERGY

Eating away from home can be a problem if you have a severe food allergy. The risk seems to be greater in some establishments, depending on the range of food to which you are allergic. The following is an example of these risks for someone with an allergy to peanut/nut and their derivatives. The risk can be greater when eating in Oriental restaurants because:

- Foods often contain more ingredients.
- Nuts and peanuts tend to be used more than in Western-style cooking.
- Ingredients may be 'hidden' within a dish and therefore are not recognised.
- A strong-flavoured dish can mask the taste of the individual ingredients (including any nuts).
- A spicy food can mask the initial sensation of an allergic reaction.

- Language problems may hinder understanding between the person with the allergy and the restaurant staff.
- Nut and peanut allergy is rare in Oriental countries, which can result in a poor understanding of the problem in Oriental establishments.

15
Cross-contamination

'Cross-contamination' is what happens when allergens are transferred from one food or food ingredient to another. In a very few instances this may result in a previously safe food becoming unsafe. If you have a severe food allergy and eat this food, thinking it is safe, you may well develop an allergic reaction. This chapter considers some of the issues.

Cross-contamination is a significant issue, but unfortunately not one that is understood by many of the general, non-allergic, community. It can happen in a wide range of circumstances, but occurs most commonly during food manufacturing and food preparation. Another type of cross-contamination occurs when food allergens are transferred not to another food but to an object or person. The list given in the section 'Out and about' is included because it may explain why, for example, you always get an itchy face after using a phone you share with a colleague.

FOOD MANUFACTURE

Food manufacturers are now much more aware of food allergy and the importance of labelling their products clearly. This is discussed in Chapter 9. They are also improving their manufacturing practices to prevent accidental cross-contamination. Some people feel that this has led to the over-use of 'may contain' labelling, which has reduced dietary choices even further.

FOOD PREPARATION

This includes food prepared at home – over which you probably have at least some control – and food prepared elsewhere.

Shopping
Many aspects of shopping can lead to cross-contamination. For example:

- Delicatessen bags may have been handled by assistants touching foods that you are allergic to.

- Food obtained from a bakery, butcher or delicatessen, because foods are not wrapped.

- Food handlers' hands may be contaminated with an allergen and then used to touch your food.

- Handling other people's food to which you are allergic. The food may even be on the outside of an unopened packet because another packet has split and spilled its contents.

- Supermarket conveyor belts may have had food allergens spilled on them and not been cleaned thoroughly.

Some of these examples may seem extreme, but they could cause a reaction.

In the kitchen

Look out particularly for the following.

- Utensils and work surfaces that are not thoroughly clean (e.g. a grater that has cheese stuck in it and you are allergic to dairy).

- Odd-shaped containers that are hard to get thoroughly clean.

- Ovens with burnt-on food which then falls onto your food.

- Cooking oil that has been used for frying many different food items, including some to which you are allergic.

- Flour or other packets having been handled by someone whose hands are contaminated with a food to which you are allergic.

- Spillages in the fridge: food to which you are allergic may spill onto your food. (For example, milk kept on the top shelf could spill onto the food below.)

- Used spoons and knives put back in a sugar bowl, marmalade jar, butter dish or coffee jar.

- Inadequate washing of ingredients (e.g. a tomato from a self-service container might have been handled by others).

- Inadequate handwashing before and between food preparation.

Points for good practice include:

- As a general rule, rinsing and then automatic dishwashing is more likely to remove food allergens than is manual dishwashing.

- Cloths harbour food allergens; replace cloths regularly and/or use disposables.

- Used chopping boards will also retain allergen contamination.

- Good handwashing using soap and water is effective in removing food allergens.

- Additional use of antibacterial handwashes is also effective in helping to remove food allergens.

MY CHECKLIST TO PREVENT CROSS-CONTAMINATION

☐ I always use gloves when I go anywhere near food to which I am allergic.

☐ I always wash fresh fruit, salad and vegetables before eating them.

☐ I never drink from a cup/glass or use cutlery/crockery unless it has been thoroughly washed.

☐ I never kiss someone without making sure that they haven't recently eaten the foods that I am allergic to.

☐ I never eat (suitable) foods from a buffet unless I can take mine first.

☐ I always inform anyone catering for me about the risk of cross-contamination, giving them plenty of notice.

☐ I always offer to take my own food to social events or make myself available to help during preparation when others are nervous about catering for my needs.

☐ I never risk eating anything that I suspect may be contaminated with food that is unsafe for me.

☐ I always carry my medication and action plan for treatment, just in case cross-contamination occurs.

Eating

The main risks of cross-contamination when you are eating arise from:

- Drinking from someone else's cup.

- Using someone else's cutlery.

- Eating a normally safe food that has been placed by food that is unsafe for you (e.g. eating grapes from a dish that also contains cheese if you are allergic to dairy).

It is essential that caterers preparing food for someone with a severe allergy understand the issues of cross-contamination. Unless you advise them about this, they probably won't realise that only a minute quantity of an allergenic food can trigger a life-threatening reaction. Never assume that a catering establishment will know about all the issues regarding food allergies. Your specific needs should be clearly written down and talked through with the person who will be preparing and serving your food.

PERSONAL CONTACT

You might react with an itchy rash in the following circumstances or contacts.

- Kissing, especially on the lips or cheeks.

- Pet foods, which can be transferred onto pets' fur if they lick themselves and you then stroke or cuddle them.

- Shaking hands.

- Vomit, if the baby or person has consumed anything that contains food that you are allergic to.

I am sure you can think of many, many more, especially those that are pertinent to *your* allergy.

A good way to ensure that you don't inadvertently expose yourself to the possibility of cross-contamination is to have a checklist. You may find the one given on the previous page helpful, and perhaps you can add to it.

Enjoying Life

16
Holidays and Travelling

Getting away from it all is an important part of life. We all need a break from our routine, and benefit from the rest, relaxation and recharging the spirit, as well as a bit of indulgence, too! This chapter tells you about options that are available to you when deciding on a holiday, whether in the UK or abroad. The information will also be useful if you are travelling on business.

TRAVELLING OR HOLIDAYING IN THE UK

Much of Chapter 14 ('Eating Away from Home') applies when you are travelling in the UK or staying somewhere on holiday.

Bed and breakfast (B&B) and guest houses

Vegan guest houses are by definition free of egg, fish, shellfish, meat and milk. (Vegetarian guest houses will not usually be egg- and milk-free.) If you have a milk or egg allergy, it should be completely safe to go to a 100% vegan guest house. Do be aware, though, that some vegan establishments have eggs and cow's milk available for their non-vegan guests. It may still be safe to stay there if these foods are kept separately, with no risk of cross-contamination.

Organisations that can supply details of places to stay and eat include:

- Action Against Allergy (contact details in Appendix 1), who will provide a list on request.
- Allergy Action website (see Appendix 2).
- Coeliac UK (details in Appendix 1), who have a list of accommodation and holiday places to stay where the proprietors or a member of the family are coeliac and they are used to cooking gluten- and wheat-free food. Many of them are also happy to cater for other special diets.
- Vegan Society (details in Appendix 1).

- 'Eating out and holiday accommodation' section in Appendix 3.

See also the website of Foodsmatter (see Appendix 2) for links to other sites with this information.

When you find a place where you feel confident, tell the Anaphylaxis Campaign, Allergy UK and Action Against Allergy about it, so that others can enjoy the facilities with confidence, too. And, of course, use it again yourself!

TRAVELLING OR HOLIDAYING ABROAD

You might think that it is impossible to eat safely and confidently when you are away from your own kitchen and in a foreign country but this is not so. If you take on board the following advice, you will minimise the risks.

It is, of course, essential to be fully prepared. You can do this by reducing the number of risks but you should also plan what to do if there is an emergency. (If you need a referral to an allergy specialist in European countries outside the UK, you should seek a doctor who is a member of the European Academy of Allergy and Clinical Immunology.)

Reducing the risk to prevent an allergic reaction
Well in advance of your holiday, obtain translation cards that explain your allergy in the language of the country (or countries) that you are travelling through or to. You can buy these from Allergy UK, the Anaphylaxis Campaign, Kidsaware or the Yellow Cross Company (contact details in Appendix 1).

I strongly recommend that you also obtain a letter from your GP stating that you are carrying medication and why. Show the letter to customs officials if there are any queries, which should prevent the possibility of your medication causing problems or being seized by them. This is especially important if you are carrying adrenaline because of the needle.

Travelling by air, sea or Channel tunnel
If you are travelling by aeroplane or any other mode of transport where food is provided, it is often possible to order a special meal (e.g. milk-free, nut-free, wheat-free). *Beware*, though, as these meals may not be what they claim, and eating them could have serious conse-

quences if you cannot get to medical care quickly. It is often easier and safer to take food that you have prepared yourself for these journeys.

If you are travelling in a group, make sure that all members of your party know about your allergy. If you are travelling alone, be sure to carry identification that will warn others of your allergy in the event that you are unable to tell them. In either case, also tell a member of the crew about your allergy.

Carry all medication in your hand luggage for easy accessibility. Do not place it in a bag that could get lost or mislaid.

If you are travelling by aeroplane and are allergic to nuts, phone the airline and request a nut-free flight. Many airlines now have a specific policy for nut-free travel. Some people have reported that they have suffered an allergic reaction while travelling on an aircraft. The cause is thought to be the free peanut snacks distributed to all passengers from the beverages trolley. When the packets are opened, the peanut dust gets into the air and is circulated and recirculated around the aircraft cabin. The Anaphylaxis Campaign has contacted a number of airlines to ask if they are willing to remove the peanut snacks from a flight if adequate notice is given; many say they will.

Arriving at your destination

As soon as you reach your destination, find out how to use the telephone so you are prepared if an emergency arises. Learning how to call a doctor and an ambulance are your priorities. Alternatively, take your mobile phone so that you have access to immediate telephone contact. (Make sure that you can use it abroad!) If you decide to take your mobile phone, it would be a good idea to programme the local 'emergency' numbers into it at the start of your holiday. They include the hospital, the doctor, a taxi company, your holiday rep (if you have one) and the proprietor or manager of your accommodation.

Find out where the nearest hospital is. It may be useful to contact the hospital at the beginning of the holiday to tell them where you are staying and what your requirements might be. Then, if an emergency does occur, all parties are well informed. You may be happier to find a hospital that has a comparable standard of healthcare to the UK.

Accommodation

If you are at risk of a severe reaction, it is probably wise to choose accommodation where you are in control of the food preparation. Choose either self-catering accommodation, so that you can prepare your own food, or catered accommodation where you are completely confident that the chef understands and is prepared to cater for your special needs.

Self-catering is probably the best option, because you are completely in control of the food that you are eating. With a kitchen of your own you can explore local markets and enjoy all the local fresh produce. However, a major part of a holiday is often the welcome escape from the domestic chores, so self-catering may not appeal to you. (If you are abroad on business, you may not have time to shop and cook!) However, many hotels now have rooms with basic kitchen facilities. Using these, you can prepare your own meals but still dine with others who are eating the hotel food. They can enjoy not having to cook while knowing that you can all enjoy eating together without worrying about your allergy.

You may prefer to choose a holiday with a representative (holiday rep) who has a good living and working knowledge of the country you are visiting. It would be advisable to make sure they have written details of your medical condition and any action plan that you have formulated. Take their mobile phone number if they have one so that they can be contacted without delay if the need arises.

Food issues on holiday
Preferably choose a holiday destination where the locals and you can understand one another and where food labelling regulations and allergy awareness are comparable to the UK (see Chapter 9).

Avoid any situations that have triggered an allergic reaction in the past. And never eat or drink anything unless you are completely confident that it is safe to do so.

Preparing food yourself

- Take your own food that you have prepared to your destination. Do not risk taking any new foods that you have not tried before.
- Ensure that all utensils in your self-catering apartment are scrupulously clean. This includes the fridge, cooker and grill pan.
- On arrival, check that the cooker hob and oven are working satisfactorily. If they are not, you may wish to change rooms or put in a request for them to be fixed as a matter of urgency.
- Take advantage of fresh foods from the local markets. Perhaps you could try to make some dishes similar to those at the local

restaurants so that you don't feel left out. (See also Chapter 13, 'Eating In'.)

- Always take your own food on days out so that you are not tempted to eat food that may not be safe for you.

Food prepared by others

If you do decide to eat out, make sure that you take translations and always check ingredients and preparation methods if they are not made clear on the menu. Always speak to the chef direct rather than via the waiter. If the chef is too busy to speak to you, he is probably too busy to take on board what you are trying to tell him so it is advisable to go elsewhere.

Most holidays involve alcohol, perhaps including the occasional cocktail. If you are having a cocktail, make sure that the shaker has been thoroughly washed, as otherwise it may contain traces of allergen. Even better – choose something else, such as a glass of wine or a bottled or canned soft drink.

Avoid drinks that have fruit added, because the boards and knives may be contaminated with food allergens. Think carefully before you have ice cubes. Although it is rare for them to be the cause of an allergic reaction, it *is* possible. Those from an ice-making machine are more likely to be safe than those made in a fridge.

If you are allowing someone else to cater for you, always double-check and confirm in writing that you both have the same understanding of your requirements and that they will be able to meet your special needs. Take a copy of the letter with you on your holiday, in case they renege on their promises. (See also Chapter 14, 'Eating Away from Home'.)

PLANNING FOR AN EMERGENCY

- Make sure that you have adequate medication in case you need it for self-administration. Not doing so could have fatal consequences. Carry this medication at all times as well as ID and an action plan on the preferred procedure for administration. This will be especially important if you are unable to administer it yourself. (See also Chapter 5, 'Your Anaphylaxis Contingency Plan'.)
- Carry an action plan in case of emergencies. Try role-playing this to ensure that everyone who might be involved understands

what to do and is confident to implement the plan swiftly and efficiently in an emergency. You may wish to get medical help when writing the action plan or have it checked over when you have written it – ask your GP or your doctor at the allergy clinic.

- Make sure that the action plan can be located immediately by all members of your party and that they know how use it.
- You must locate the nearest hospital and know how to get there quickly if you need treatment. To speed up the treatment, you should have details of the nature of your allergy and the action required if you have a serious reaction. If you are going abroad, make sure that you have clear translations.
- Obtain adequate travel insurance. It is essential that you tell the sales assistant about your allergy and ensure it is documented on the application form; otherwise, you may not be covered if you make a claim.
- If you are travelling through or to European Union countries, obtain the European Health Insurance Card (EHIC), which has replaced the form E111. The application form can be obtained from the Post Office or from the EHIC Application office (contact details in Appendix 1). Remember to carry it with your other travel documents.
- If you are worried that your medication will deteriorate because you are going to a country with a hot climate, you may wish to purchase a small insulated bag in which to keep it. The Yellow Cross Company and Kidsaware (contact details in Appendix 1) have various carry-bags.
- Carry spare copies of your guidance notes with you to hand to chefs (have them laminated so that they can be cleaned easily if they get splashed in a busy kitchen).
- You could take this book with you as a reference guide, especially if others you are travelling with are not used to your allergy. Two other publications that you may find useful are the *Travellers Guide to Health*, which is a Department of Health booklet, and *Allergies: answers at your fingertips* (see Appendix 3).

As well as all the above points, make sure you read – or re-read – Chapter 14 ('Eating Away from Home').

OTHER ISSUES

Taking new medication and going to the dentist when you are abroad are two scenarios to talk through with your NHS allergy specialist before you go. Do not agree to use any new medication or injections while abroad unless you are sure it is safe for you to do so.

SUMMARY

Below is a checklist for you to work through to make sure that you have done everything possible to ensure a relaxed and safe holiday.

CHECKLIST FOR TRAVELLING

☐ I have asked my doctor:
  – for a brief medical history to take with me,
  – to help me formulate or check my action plan for emergency use.

☐ I have obtained a letter from my GP regarding my carrying adrenaline injector(s).

☐ I have obtained a translation describing my allergy and my emergency action plan and have extra copies to give to key people.

☐ I have obtained the name, address and phone number of a doctor at my holiday destination.

☐ I have obtained the name, address and phone number of the hospital nearest to where I will be staying.

☐ I have obtained the emergency phone number of the country I'm going to (e.g. 999 in the UK).

☐ I have arranged adequate medical holiday insurance, advising the insurer about my allergy.

☐ I have noted my National Insurance number and obtained my European Health Insurance Card from the post office.

☐ I have obtained an extra supply of my medication.

☐ I have packed my health insurance details.

☐ I have made a copy of all the documents listed above, and will carry a set with me at all times on holiday and leave another in my room.

☐ I will carry my medication at all times.

☐ I have a list of people at home who should be contacted in the event of an emergency.

ENGLISH	FRENCH	GERMAN	SPANISH
Almonds	Amandes	Mandeln	Almendra
Bananas	Bananes	Bananen	Plátanos
Beans	Haricots	Bohnen	Habas
Brazil nuts	Noix du Brésil	Brasilnüsse/Paranüsse	Nueces del Brasil
Cashews	Noix d'acajou	Cashewnüsse	Anacardos
Chestnuts	Châtaignes/Marrons	Kastanien	Castañas
Chocolate	Cacao/Chocolat	Schokolade	Chocolate
Coconut	Noix de Coco	Kokosnuß	Coco
Eggs	Oeufs	Eier	Huevos
Fish	Poisson	Fisch	Pez
Hazelnuts	Noisettes	Haselnüsse	Avellanas
Lentils	Lentilles	Linsen	Lentejas
Milk	Lait	Milch	Leche
Mushrooms	Champignons	Champignons	Setas u hongos
Nut oils	Huiles de noix	Nußöle	Aceite de nueces
Nuts	Noix	Nüsse	Nueces
Oranges	Oranges	Orangen	Naranjas
Peaches	Pêches	Pfirsiche	Duraznos
Peanuts	Huile d'arachide/ Cacahuètes/Arachides	Erdnüsse	Cacahuetes
Peas	Petits pois	Erbsen	Guisantes
Pecan nuts	Pacanes	Pekannüsse	Pacanas
Pesto sauce	Sauce au basilic et aux pignons	Pestosoße	Salsa de hierbas/ aceite
Pine nuts	Pignes	Pinienkerne	Piñas
Pulses	Légumes à gousse/ légumes secs	Hülsenfrüchte	Legumbres
Seafood	Fruits de mer	Meeresfrüchte	Mariscos
Sesame seeds	Graines de sésame	Sesamsamen	Sesamo
Soya	Soya/soja (Graines de soja/farine de soja)	Soya	Soja
Strawberries	Fraises	Erdbeeren	Fresas
Tomatoes	Tomates	Tomaten	Tomates
Walnuts	Noix	Walnüsse	Nueces de nogal
Wheat	Blé	Weizen	Trigo
Yeast	Levure	Hefe	Levadura

These translations were provided by native speakers for the benefit of those at risk.

ITALIAN	GREEK	DUTCH	PORTUGUESE
Mandorle	Αμύγδαλο	Amandelen	Amêndoas
Banane	Μπανάνα	Bananen	Bananas
Fagioli	Φασόλια	Bonen	Feijão
Castagne del Brasile	Βραζιλιάνικα καρύδια	Braziliaanse noten	Castanha-do-pará
Anacardi	Κάσιους	Cashew noten	Castanha de caju
Castagne	Κάστανα	Kastanjes	Castanhas
Cacao, cioccolata	Σοκολάτα	Chocolade	Chocolate
Cocco	Καρύδα	Kokosnoot	Coco
Uova	Αυγά	Eieren	Ovos
Pesce	Ψάρι	Vis	Peixe
Nocciole	Φουντούκια	Hazelnoten	Avelás
Lenticchie	Φακές	Linzen	Lentilhas
Latte	Γάλα	Melk	Leite
Funghi	Μανιτάρια	Paddestoelen	Cogumelos
Olii di noci, arachidi e simili	Λάδι από ξηρούς καρπούς	Noten Olie	Azeite de nozes
Noci, nocciole, arachidi e frutti secchi	Ξηροί καρποί	Noten	Fruta seca
Arance	Πορτοκάλια	Sinaasappels	Laranjas
Pesche	Ροδάκινα	Perziken	Pêssegos
Arachidi, noccioline	Φυστίκια αράπικα	Pindas	Amendoim
Piselli	Μπιζέλια, αρακάς	Erwten	Ervilhas
Pecan, noce americana	Πέκαν καρύδια	Pecan noten	Pecan
Salsa al pesto	Σάλτσα με βασιλικό	Pesto (basilicumsaus)	Molho das ervas e azeite
Pinoli	Κουκουνάρια	Pijnboompitten	Pinho
Legumi	Όσπρια	Peulvruchten	Legumes
Frutti di mare/ pesce in generale	Οστρακοειδή, θαλασσινά	Vis	Mariscos
Semi de sesame	Σουσάμι	Sesamzaad	Sementes de sesamo
Soya	Σόγια	Soja	Soya
Fragole	Φράουλες	Aardbeien	Morangos
Pomodori	Ντομάτες	Tomaten	Tomates
Noci	Καρύδια	Walnoten	Nogueiras
Grano	Σιτάρι	Tarwe	Trigo
Lievito	Προζύμι, μαγιά	Gist	Levedura

© 2005 Hazel Gowland www.allergyaction.org. Reproduced with permission

TRANSLATIONS OF COMMON FOOD ALLERGIES

17
Help for People on Special Diets

Having to use 'special diet' foods and other allergen-free products can be expensive. They usually cost more than ordinary food and ingredients. This chapter outlines some ways that may help you financially or just gives some useful advice.

FREE PRESCRIPTIONS

Even if you are not entitled to free prescriptions for the medication you need for an allergy, it may be useful to know the criteria to qualify for this in case your circumstances change.

You are entitled to exemption from prescription charges if you:

- are a permanent resident in a nursing/residential home (at least partly funded by the local authority),
- are a war-disabled pensioner,
- are aged 60 or over,
- have a child under the age of one year,
- are on a low income (holding certificate HC2),
- are pregnant,
- are under 16, or under 19 and in full-time education,
- have:
  - a continuing disability,
  - a permanent fistula requiring continuous surgical dressing or appliance,
  - diabetes insipidus or other hypopituitarism,
  - diabetes mellitus and are taking medication for it,
  - epilepsy requiring continuous anti-convulsive therapy,
  - a form of hypoadrenalism (including Addison's disease),
  - hypoparathyroidism,
  - myasthenia gravis,
  - myxoedema (underactive thyroid).

In addition, if you or your partner receives the following state benefits, you are automatically entitled to free prescriptions:

- income-based JobSeekers Allowance,
- Income Support,
- Family Credit,
- NHS Tax Credit Exemption certificate,
- Pension Credit guarantee credit.

Other people in receipt of means-tested benefits may also be eligible. If you think that you might be eligible, consult leaflet HC11 – *Are You Entitled to Help with Health Costs?* – available at main post offices and social security offices and from many GP surgeries and pharmacy/chemist shops.

People who are exempt from paying prescription charges are now asked to provide proof of their exemption when they collect their prescription. Failure to do so may mean that they have to pay the prescription charge.

PREPAYMENT CERTIFICATE ('SEASON TICKET') FOR PRESCRIPTIONS

If you need lots of prescriptions, it may save money in the long run to pre-pay the prescription charges with a prepayment certificate, often called a season ticket. This can be purchased for a period of four months or one year. Once the initial fee has been paid, all prescription charges will be free for the chosen period. If you are likely to need six or more items in four months or 15 or more in a year, it is probably worth your while getting a 'season ticket'. Further information about them is available from most pharmacy/chemist shops, GP surgeries and post office counters (ask for form FP95).

OVER-THE-COUNTER MEDICINES

Many medicines on prescription are also available over the counter – without a prescription – direct from the pharmacy/chemist shop or pharmacy department in the supermarket. Sometimes the cost will be less than the prescription charge. To ensure that you are getting medicines in the most economical way, it is useful to check this out with the pharmacist.

NON-COW'S MILK FORMULA ON PRESCRIPTION

Babies who are unable to tolerate cow's milk formula are entitled to get an alternative on prescription from the GP. Because babies are exempt from paying prescription charges, this will be free.

GLUTEN-FREE PRODUCTS

Many gluten-free products (basic food items such as bread, flour and pasta) are prescribable by the GP for people with coeliac disease. Occasionally, GPs agree to prescribe these products for someone with another food allergy or intolerance. This is more likely to happen if the person has seen a dietitian or been to an allergy clinic where a formal diagnosis has been made.

WHOLE-EGG REPLACER

Whole-egg replacer is available on prescription. It can be used as a replacement for eggs in recipes, adding variety to the diet. (See also 'Egg-free diet' in Chapter 10.)

STATE BENEFITS

Social Fund

This is a state benefit that is usually accessed in relation to a special need. For example, if a washing machine or vacuum cleaner is required to keep your house dust-mite-free for a child with severe eczema, or an oven is required to cook special dietary products in, this fund may pay for it. Details can be obtained from your local social security office.

Disability Living Allowance (DLA), care component

This is available for anyone under 65 who needs extra personal care in the long term. For example, the extra care for a child with eczema who requires time-consuming treatments such as wet wraps or for the extra time that is required to shop and cook for a special diet. The care part of the DLA has three rates, depending on the amount of care the person needs. All cases are judged individually, and success in obtaining DLA for an allergy-related condition varies.

Invalid Care Allowance

If someone is receiving DLA at the upper or middle rate, their main carer may be entitled to claim Invalid Care Allowance if they are providing at least 35 hours of care a week.

Claiming state benefits

To claim any of the above benefits, first get the relevant leaflets from your local social security office (the phone number will be in your telephone directory).

If your claim is unsuccessful, you can then appeal against the decision. To do this you will require medical reports from your GP and hospital consultant. Advice from the local Citizens Advice Bureau (CAB) may also be useful in preparing your case.

NON-FINANCIAL SOURCES OF HELP WHEN ON A SPECIAL DIET

There are many ways to find help and advice about special diets. They include:

- Action Against Allergy,
- allergy specialist,
- allergy support group,
- Allergy UK,
- Anaphylaxis Campaign,
- Baby Milk Action,
- community children's nurse,
- dietitian,
- food manufacturers,
- GP,
- health fairs/shows,
- health visitor,
- healthfood shops,
- internet websites,
- library,
- paediatric dietitian,
- school nurse,
- special diet cookbooks,
- supermarkets,
- Vegan Society.

And many, many more – add your own suggestions below so that you can refer to the list in times of need. (Contact details of the organisations listed above can be found in Appendix 1.)

18
Career and Leisure Choices

Depending on the nature of your food allergy and any other allergies that you may have, it would probably be useful to consider issues that could affect your choices of career and hobbies. It is sensible to look at this factor before you start training for a career in one of these areas.

FOOD ALLERGY

If you have a severe food allergy, the following careers may prove to be unsuitable choices:

- bakery,
- chef/catering staff,
- childcare/nanny,
- cocktail bar worker,
- food factory worker,
- food handler,
- food shop worker,
- kitchen hand,
- waiter/waitress.

OTHER ALLERGY

Many people with severe food allergies often also have asthma, eczema or hay-fever. In view of this, it would be useful to bear this in mind when planning to invest time and finances in career and leisure choices. The following are examples of careers that may need extra thought beforehand:

- carpenter,
- carpet seller,

- cement worker,
- cleaner,
- factory worker (some),
- florist,
- hairdresser,
- jockey,
- nurse,
- pub worker,
- vet/veterinary nurse,
- waiter/waitress,
- washer-upper.

OTHER CHOICES

Don't worry if the lists seem rather long. It is not that these careers are totally unsuitable, just that you may experience difficulties and would need to find alternative ways of doing some things.

Here are some preferable career choices:

- actor,
- administrator,
- artist,
- author,
- dancer,
- designer,
- dietitian,
- doctor,
- engineer,
- journalist,
- lawyer,
- lecturer,
- newsreader,
- police officer,
- receptionist,

- salesperson,
- secretary,
- teacher,

etc., etc., etc.!

Although many jobs require the use of gloves traditionally made of latex, this can be overcome with non-latex gloves.

LEISURE

There are certain leisure activities that might be unsuitable if you have a severe food allergy or are allergic to grass, pollen, animal fur, dust and other allergens. It is useful to make your leisure choices with this in mind. Think about the relevant choices and try them out. Whatever you do, though, *enjoy yourself and have some fun*!

There is absolutely no reason why you cannot enjoy a fulfilling work and social life because of your severe food allergy, or any other allergy. Being informed and understanding your allergy and knowing what action to take if a severe reaction is triggered are the key to successfully putting it to the back of your mind and getting on with the things that matter to you in life.

I hope that this book will have helped you to enjoy life and food safely despite having a severe food allergy.

Glossary

Terms in *italic* in the definitions are also given in the Glossary

acute short term, intense; the opposite of *chronic*

adrenaline adrenaline (also called epinephrine) is a hormone produced by the adrenal glands when we exercise or are feeling afraid or stressed. It acts on the blood vessels (arteries and veins) to maintain normal blood pressure and circulation. In *anaphylaxis* it is given as an emergency injection to do just this, to reverse the symptoms of the reaction

allergen a substance – usually a protein molecule (e.g. nut protein, milk protein, egg protein) – that can trigger the body's *immune system* to produce *antibodies* and thereby cause an *allergic reaction*. (See also *antigen*)

allergic reaction an immune reaction involving a specific type of *antibody* – immunoglobulin E (IgE)

allergic rhinitis *inflammation* of the lining of the nose, caused by an *allergic reaction*

allergy an abnormal or inappropriate reaction of the body's *immune system* to a substance (an *allergen)* that would normally be harmless

anaphylactic shock/anaphylaxis a sudden, severe *allergic reaction* to an *allergen* that can be life-threatening; if untreated, it can lead to dizziness, shortness of breath, wheezing, palpitations, a serious drop in blood pressure and collapse

angioedema the presence of fluid in the deep layers of the skin (the dermis), particularly of the face, eyes, lips, tongue and throat, as a result of an *allergic reaction*

antibodies produced by the *immune system* in response to a foreign substance, antibodies circulate in the blood serum and help to fight infection and foreign elements called *antigens*. (See also *immunoglobulins*)

antigen a substance capable of inducing an immune response. (See also *allergen*)

antihistamines drugs that block the action of *histamine*

Arachis hypogaea the botanical name for the peanut plant

arachis oil peanut oil

asthma a *chronic* lung disease in which *inflammation* of the airways and twitchiness of the airway wall muscles make it difficult to move air in and out of the lungs, and cause the symptoms of wheezing, coughing and tightness of the chest, making it difficult to breathe

atopic/atopy an inherited tendency to develop an *allergy* or allergies such as *asthma*, *eczema* and hay-fever

bronchi the branching airways that carry air to and from the lungs

challenge test a test that involves a substance (e.g. a suspect food) being given in increasing amounts to see if an *allergic reaction* will occur, and, if so, at what level of exposure

chronic persisting for a long time; the opposite of *acute*

circulatory collapse the blood vessels in the tissues (the capillaries) dilate and become more leaky. Because of this, less blood returns to the heart to be pumped round the body, blood pressure falls and oxygen delivery to the tissues becomes less efficient. Eventually, oxygen delivery is so poor and the blood pressure is so low that the circulatory system collapses and so does the person

complementary therapies treatments that may be used in addition to conventional medicine. Popular examples are acupuncture, aromatherapy, homoeopathy and osteopathy

conjunctivitis *inflammation* of the conjunctiva, which is a delicate membrane that lines the eyelids and covers the eyeballs; it causes itchy, watering red eyes and is often associated with *allergic rhinitis*

corticosteroids a group of chemicals produced naturally in the body by the adrenal glands, which are vital for the body's defences against infection and stress. They can also be manufactured (and are often called 'steroids'). Used as anti-inflammatory drugs they suppress the body's *immune system* and thereby dampen the inflammatory over-reaction. They come as creams, inhalants, nasal sprays, tablets and eye drops

COT Committee on Toxicity of Chemicals in Foods, Consumer Products and the Environment: a committee of independent experts that advises the Government

cross-reactivity associations between allergies due to common *allergens*. For example, some people who are allergic to latex get symptoms from eating banana, avocado or kiwi fruit

crude oil unrefined oil that may contain sufficient quantities of protein to induce an *allergic reaction*

desensitisation see *immunotherapy*

dietitian a professional with medical training in using diet as a therapy for illness and who gives advice about all aspects of food and diet

eczema a *chronic* inflammatory condition of the skin that makes it itchy. In mild cases the skin is dry and scaly but it can become red, blistered and weepy if severe

epinephrine see *adrenaline*

exacerbate make worse

food allergy an exaggerated immune response triggered by a specific food

food and symptom diary a diary in which you list all the food and drinks you have consumed and any symptoms experienced during a set period

gluten a protein found in wheat, barley, oats and rye

ground nut a member of the *Leguminosae* family that grows in the ground (e.g. peanut). Other members of this family include peas, beans and lentils

histamine a chemical released by the body during an *allergic reaction*. Histamine causes *inflammation* and the symptoms of *allergy*.

hives another name for *urticaria*

hydrocortisone see *corticosteroids*

idiopathic a description that means 'of unknown cause'. When applied to a disease or a disorder, it means that the cause of the problem is either not known or has not yet been identified, for example idiopathic *anaphylaxis*

immune system the body's complex system that protects us from infections and foreign substances. In allergic people the *immune system* over-reacts to agents that are harmless to non-allergic people

immunoglobulin E (IgE) an *antibody* that is involved in *allergy* and *anaphylaxis*

immunotherapy a form of allergy treatment in which gradually increasing doses of an *allergen* are administered until the allergic person can tolerate exposure without developing major symptoms. Also called 'desensitisation'

incidence the number of new cases of a disease that occur in a defined population during a particular time

inflammation the reaction of the body to infection, injury or disease. Its purpose is to protect the body from further harm. In allergy the inappropriate inflammation damages the body rather than protects it

intolerance when the body reacts inappropriately – but without producing *immunoglobulin E* (IgE) – to a particular substance. An example is lactose intolerance

lactose a sugar found in animal milks (including human milk). The term is most commonly used to refer to the sugar in cow's milk

Leguminosae the pea and bean (legume) family of foods, of which the peanut and soya bean are part

mast cells cells containing *histamine*, which is released during an *allergic reaction*

mucosa the mucus membrane that lines many parts (the hollow organs) of the body, such as the gut and the airways

nettle rash another name for *urticaria*

open challenge a test for food allergy in which both the doctor doing the testing and the person being tested know what foods are being given

oral allergy syndrome an *allergic reaction* to certain proteins found in a variety of fruit, vegetables and nuts

osteoporosis thinning of the bones as a result of overall loss of calcium from the body

pareve a category of kosher food: it contains neither meat nor dairy products, nor their derivatives, and it is not processed on equipment that has processed products containing meat

patch test a skin test for diagnosing which *allergens* someone is allergic to; it is particularly useful for contact *eczema*, or dermatitis

prevalence a measure of the number of people in the population with a particular medical condition at any one time. For example, if we say that the current prevalence of severe food allergy is 2%, we mean that 2% of the population has a severe food allergy at this moment

prophylactic something given as a protective or preventative measure

provocation test see *challenge test*

rash a skin eruption

RAST (radio-allergosorbent test) a specific diagnostic blood test for detecting *immunoglobulin E* (IgE) *antibodies* against a suspected *allergen*

rescue medication medication (e.g. *antihistamine* or *adrenaline*) taken in the event of a severe reaction to an *allergen*

rhinitis *inflammation* of the lining of the nose. The symptoms include a blocked nose, runny nose and sneezing

skin-prick test a diagnostic test used to identify which *allergens* someone is allergic to. A drop of a liquid preparation of the concentrated allergen is applied to the skin on the back or on the inside of the forearm, and the skin is then pricked through the droplet. The response is measured after 10–15 minutes. The procedure is painless, gives rapid results and is probably the most commonly used and most informative allergy test

specific IgE test *see* RAST

symptom diary a record of your symptoms and the factors thought to be causing them. People who have an *allergy* problem are often completely well on the day on which they see their doctor, so it is therefore very useful for a doctor to see a detailed record of how serious the problem is, what form it takes and what might be provoking it

texture milestones stages at which babies start eating foods with certain textures; e.g. pureed, mashed, lumpy.

tree nut a nut that grows on a tree (e.g. Brazil nut, hazelnut, macadamia nut, pecan, walnut, almond)

triggers or **trigger factors** popular name for anything that may bring on allergic symptoms or make them worse

urticaria swelling of the superficial layers of the skin, usually as a result of an allergic reaction. The characteristic itchy lumps (also called 'hives' or 'nettle rash') last for only a few hours

weal a bump in the skin which can be a response to an allergen

ABBREVIATIONS

AAA	Action Against Allergy
AFAD	Association for Allergic Disorders
BNF	British Nutrition Foundation
BSACI	British Society of Allergy and Clinical Immunology
CAB	Citizens Advice Bureau
COT	Committee on Toxicity of Chemicals in Foods, Consumer Products and the Environment
DfES	Department for Education and Skills
DOH	Department of Health
FAC	Food Advisory Committee
FSA	Food Standards Agency
INCI	International Nomenclature of Cosmetic Ingredients
NICE	National Institute for Health and Clinical Excellence
SCOPA	Seed Crushers and Oil Producers Association
SPT	skin-prick test

Appendix 1
Useful Addresses

The **Anaphylaxis Campaign** is a registered charity with the aim of helping people with severe allergies obtain a better quality of life.

It has a wide range of products and information, including:

- information packs for schools, caterers, GPs, dietitians, teenagers, pre-school groups and youth movements

- fact sheets on different sorts of allergies plus frequently asked questions, challenge testing, translations of Latin, and airlines and travel

- booklets (listed in Appendix 3)

- videos and DVDs (listed in Appendix 3)

- links to their sister sites for schools and caterers (see Appendix 2)

The Anaphylaxis Campaign also arranges meetings and workshops around the UK: support group meetings, parent workshops, youth workshops, family fun days and public awareness meetings.

For contact details, see the entry on the next page.

USEFUL ORGANISATIONS

Action Against Allergy
PO Box 278
Twickenham
Middx TW1 4QQ
Tel: 020 8892 2711
Website: www.actionagainstallergy.co.uk
A support charity, providing information (including holiday and accommodation), suppliers list, newsletter advice on specialist referrals. Send s.a.e. for information.

ALK-ABELLÓ (UK)
1 Tealgate
Hungerford
Berks RG17 0YT
Tel: 01488 686 016
Website: www.epipen.co.uk
Imports and distributes the Epipen, EpiPen Junior and EpiPen Trainer in the UK. The trainer pen can be purchased directly from them.

Allergy UK
3 White Oak Square
London Road
Swanley
Kent BR8 7AG
Helpline: 01322 619898
Website: www.allergyuk.org
*Bookets, leaflets, quarterly newsletter,
support group network. A helpline for
advice and information. Provides
education courses. Lobbies government
for better services. Tests products for
allergy relief/protection.*

Anapen
see Lincoln Medical

Anaphylaxis Campaign
PO Box 275
Farnborough
Hants GU14 6SX
Helpline: 01252 542 029
Website: www.anaphylaxis.org.uk
*Set up in 1994 to spread awareness and
information about life-threatening
allergic reactions. By mid-2005 there
were 8,000 members across the UK,
most being the parents of children with
peanut/nut allergy. The Campaign
produces a range of educational news
sheets and videos. It has an extensive
support group network.*

Asthma UK
Summit House
70 Wilson Street
London EC2A 2DB
Adviceline: 08457 01 02 03
Supporter & Information Team: 020
7786 5000
Tel: 020 7786 4900
Website: www.asthma.org.uk
*Support association for people with
asthma and their families.*

Baby Milk Action
34 Trumpington Street
Cambridge CB2 1QY
Tel: 01223 464 420
Website: www.babymilkaction.org
*Produces and distributes information
and resources on infant nutrition.*

British Dietetic Association
5th floor, Charles House
148/9 Great Charles Street
Queensway
Birmingham B3 3HT
Tel: 0121 200 8080
Website: www.bda.uk.com
*National association for dietitians.
Useful allergy-related publications.
Has a special interest group for food
allergy and intolerance.*

British Nutrition Foundation
High Holborn House
52–54 High Holborn
London WC1V 6RQ
Tel: 020 7404 6504
Website: www.nutrition.org.uk
*Provides information on nutrition in the
UK.*

**British Society for Allergy and Clinical
Immunology (BSACI)**
17 Doughty Street
London WC1N 2PL
Tel: 020 7404 0278
Website: www.bsaci.org
*Aims to improve allergy services.
Website lists NHS allergy clinics in the
UK.*

Coeliac UK
PO Box 220
High Wycombe
Bucks HP11 2HS
Tel: 01494 437278
Helpline: 0870 444 8804
Website: www.coeliac.co.uk
*A registered charity that produces and
distributes useful and informative
literature on living with the coeliac
condition, including a quarterly
newsletter called* The Crossed Grain, *a
list of products available on prescription
and an annual directory listing gluten-
free manufactured foods. Regular
updates to the directory can be obtained
from them.*

**Cosmetic Toiletries & Perfumeries Association
(CTPA)**
Josaron House
5–7 John Princes Street
London W1G 0JN
Tel: 020 7491 8891
Website: www.ctpa.org.uk
*Information on the INCI names of
cosmetic ingredients, and about suitable
cosmetics, perfumes and toiletries,
depending on your allergy and what you
are trying to avoid.*

Department of Health (DoH)
Richmond House
79 Whitehall
London SW1A 2NS
Tel: 020 7210 4850
Freephone 0800 555 777
(health literature line)
Website: www.dh.gov.uk
*Produces and distributes literature
about public health, including matters
relating to food allergy and nutrition.*

DfES Publications
PO Box 5050
Sherwood Park
Annesley
Notts NG15 0DJ
Tel: 0870 000 2288
Website: www.dfes.gov.uk/publications
*Department for Education and Skills.
To obtain* Managing Medicines in
Schools and Early Years Settings *(by
DfES + Department of Health).*

EpiPen
see ALK-ABELLÓ (UK)

Food and Drink Federation (FDF)
6 Catherine Street
London WC2B 5JJ
Tel: 020 7836 2460
Website: www.fdf.org.uk
Produces annually updated Food
Allergen Advice Notes *and deals with
current food issues for food
manufacturers.*

Food Standards Agency
Aviation House
125 Kingsway
London WC2B 6NH
Tel: 020 7278 8000
Website: www.foodstandards.gov.uk
*Sets standards in relation to food issues
and ensures that these are being kept to
by food producers, distributors and
caterers. At the same address is the Food
Labelling and Standards Division,
regarding all matters relating to food
allergy and intolerance.*
  Guidance on Allergies
Management and Consumer
Information *available from 0845 606
0667 or from* foodstandards@ecgroup.uk.com

Frio UK Ltd
PO Box 10
Haverfordwest SA62 5YG
Tel: 01437 741700/741755
Website: www.friouk.com
*Manufacturer and distributor of the
FRIO-PACK, designed to keep the
EpiPen and Anapen or other medication
at a constant temperature. Particularly
useful when travelling in a hot country.*

Kidsaware
PO Box 115
Bedford MK44 2FA
Tel: 0870 220 2452
Website: www.kidsaware.com
*Awareness clothing and accessories for
babies and children with allergies: bibs,
hats, lunchboxes, tops, bags, coolbags,
ID, stickers, wristbands, and more.*

Latex Allergy Support Group
PO Box 27
Filey YO14 9YH
Helpline: 07071 225 838
(7p.m.–10p.m.)
Website: ww.lasg.co.uk
*Members receive the quarterly
newsletter, fact sheets and list of
everyday items that contain latex and
those that are latex-free. Information
and advice available on request.*

Lincoln Medical Ltd
13 Boathouse Meadow Business Park
Cherry Orchard Lane
Salisbury SP2 7LD
Tel: 0870 220 2452
Website: www.anapen.co.uk
*Distributor of the Anapen and Anapen
trainer pens.*

London Beth Din
735 High Road
London N12 0US
Tel: 020 8343 6246/6255
Website: www.kosher.org.uk
*For information about kosher food. The
Kashrut Division publishes* The Really
Jewish Food Guide.

Medic-Alert Foundation
1 Bridge Wharf
156 Caledonian Road
London N1 9UU
Tel: 020 7833 3034
Freephone: 0800 581 420
Website: www.medicalert.org.uk
*Produces a selection of identification
'jewellery' with an internationally
recognised medical symbol and 24-hour
emergency telephone number, for people
with hidden medical conditions.*

Medi-Tag
Hoopers
37 Northampton Street
Hockley
Birmingham B18 6DU
Tel: 0121 200 1616
Website: www.hoopers.org/Mediset.htm
*A division of Hoopers Healthcare
Products, Med-Tag produces
identification jewellery, including a
selection of pendants, bracelets and
watches.*

Merton Books
PO Box 279
Twickenham
Middx TW1 4XQ
Tel: 020 8892 4949
Website: www.mertonbooks.co.uk
*Publishers and stockists of a large
selection of books on allergies by mail
order. Allergy book list also available
from Action Against Allergy (which
see).*

**Midlands Asthma and Allergy Research
Association (MAARA)**
PO Box 1057
Leicester LE2 3GZ
Tel: 0116 270 7557
Website: www.maara.org
*A research and support association
offering advice and information for
people with allergies and their families.
Research (AAIR) is the Leicester
branch of MAARA (with its own
website).*

National Eczema Society
Hill House
Highgate Hill
London N19 5NA
Tel: 020 7281 3553
Helpline: 0870 241 3604
Website: www.eczema.org
*Provides information leaflets, a
newsletter and a helpline for people with
eczema and for parents of children with
eczema. A support network covers all
areas of the UK.*

National Osteoporosis Society
Camerton
Bath BA2 0PJ
Helpline: 0845 450 0230
Tel: 01761 471 771
Website: www.NOS.org.uk
*Information regarding osteoporosis, its
prevention and treatment, with a
network of local support groups. Also
has calcium information.*

Purple Kitchen Company
PO Box 1164
Beaconsfield
Buckinghamshire HP9 2WP
Tel: 01494 678688
Website: www.thepurplekitchencompany.com
*Specialises in children's cooking for 2–5
years during term time, where children
and adults learn together. Food allergies
and intolerances accommodated.
Holiday cooking classes for children aged
5–11 years. School programmes by
arrangement.*

Royal Pharmaceutical Society of Great Britain
1 Lambeth High Street
London SE1 7JN
Tel: 020 7735 9141
Website: www.rspgb.org
*Professional organisation of pharma-
cists. Publishes* Emergency First Aid:
professional standards *('the Little Red
Book').*

SOS Talisman
Tel: 0141 639 7090
Website: www.sostalisman.com
*Produces a selection of identification
jewellery available by phone or online.*

Vegan Society
Donald Watson House
7 Battle Road
St Leonards-on-Sea
East Sussex TN37 7AA
Helpline: 0845 458 8244
Tel: 01424 427 393
Website: www.vegansociety.com
*Has an excellent selection of vegan
cookery books and travel guides.
Distributor for Condomi Condoms
(milk-protein-free condoms). The
website is an excellent source about
foods and products free from milk, eggs,
animals, fish and shellfish.*

Vegetarian Guides Ltd
PO Box 2284
London W1A 5UH
Tel: 020 7254 3984
Website: www.vegetarianguides.co.uk
*Guides to vegetarian and vegan
restaurants, cafés, B&Bs, hotels, bars,
etc., in cities and countryside around the
world. Especially useful for anyone
avoiding meat, fish, eggs, milk and dairy
products.*

Yellow Cross Company Ltd
PO Box 448
Farnham
Surrey GU9 8ZU
Tel: 01252 820321
Website: www.yellowcross.co.uk
*Range of medical kit bags: thermobag,
pillpocket, schoolbag, medical
translation cards, eating-out translation
cards, personal ID tags and card, and
medical kit labels. For adults and
children.*

MANUFACTURERS AND SUPPLIERS OF SPECIAL DIET PRODUCTS

Where no contact address or
telephone number is given, ask your
local healthfood shop for details of
the product. Alternatively, contact a
distributor direct (such as Goodness
Foods, listed in the next section).

Alpro Soya
Alpro UK Ltd
Latimer Business Park
Altendiez Way
Burton Latimer
Kettering NN15 5YT
Tel: 0800 018 8180
Website: www.alprosoya.co.uk
*Range of widely available dairy-free
products: desserts, custards, yoghurts,
milks, soyafruity-cream.*

Anglesey Natural Foods Ltd
Celtic House
Gaerwen
Anglesey LL60 6HR
Tel: 01248 422 011
Website: www.quinova.co.uk
*Manufacturers of Avalon egg-free dip
and salad dressing: plain, garlic, cajun.
Also Biddy Merkins brand Vegerella
dairy-free cheese substitute (also gluten-
and soya-free and vegan). Available from
healthfood shops and distributors
Marigold Healthfoods Ltd and Suma
Wholefoods.*

Animal Aid
The Old Chapel
Bradford Street
Tonbridge
Kent TN9 1AW
Tel: 01732 364 546
Website: www.animalaid.org.uk
Organisation selling vegan wines, bars and boxes of dairy-free chocolates and fudge.

Barkat
c/o Gluten Free Foods Ltd [see below]
Gluten-free bread mixes; pizza crust and breads free from gluten, wheat, egg, milk and soya.

Blue Dragon Foods
c/o G Costa & Co. Ltd [see below]
Website: www.bluedragon.co.uk
Coconut milks, creamed coconut, coconut powder, creamy coconut; thick rice noodles; rice flour pancakes; rice vinegar, egg-free wheat noodles.

Buxton Foods Ltd
12 Harley Street
London W1G 9PG
Tel: 020 7637 5505
Website: www.buxtonfoods.com
The Stamp Collection: *dairy-free and no-added-sugar chocolate with sultana, apricot and sunflower centres. Also wheat-free pasta, bread, rolls, cookies, flours and baking mixes. Vegetable chips. Includes* Peter Rabbit Organics. *Recipes and cookbook for special diets. Available by mail order and in some supermarkets and high street shops nation-wide.*

Castle Kitchens Ltd
Castle Farm Estates
The Hollow
Washington
West Sussex RH20 3DA
Tel: 01903 891400
Website: www.castle-kitchens.com
Selection of allergen-free ready meals, available by phone and online and from some supermarkets.

Chocoreale
Vegan Store Ltd
PO Box 110
Rottingdean
Brighton BN51 9AZ
Tel: 01273 302979
Website: www.veganstore.co.uk
Supplier of organic chocolate spreads: chocolate hazelnut, chococream, chocoreale duo with vanilla swirl.

Clearspring Ltd
19A Acton Park Estate
London W3 7QE
Tel: 020 8749 1781
Website: www.clearspring.co.uk
Dairy-free products; selection of rice cakes; gluten- and wheat-free foods; Japanese sauces, sea vegetables and teas. Rice Dream: *a rice-based milk substitute; and* Imagine: *dairy-free desserts in various flavours. Available by mail order and from healthfood shops and supermarkets; also via the Goodness Direct [distributor] website.*

G Costa & Co. Ltd
Unit 6
Quarrywood Industrial Estate
Mills Road
Aylesford
Kent ME20 7NA
Tel: 01622 713 777
Customer Services: 01622 713 330
Website: www.gcosta.co.uk
Zest Foods *vegan pesto and sun-dried tomato paste. Rice noodles, rice crackers, rice vinegar, rice snacks, corn chips, egg-free wheat noodles, coconut milk*

Devon Fudge Direct
Radfords of Devon
Unit 3
2A Barton Hill Road
Torquay
Devon TQ2 8JH
Tel: 01803 316 020
Email: radfords.fudge@euphony.net
Excellent range of Radfords' assorted dairy-free coconut ice and fudge; walnut, ginger, chocolate, cherry, and rum & raisin. Available from Animal Aid, Dr Hadwen Trust and Viva!

Dietary Needs Direct
Fairfield Court Industrial Estate
Fairfield Court
Fairfield
Bromsgrove
Worcs B61 9NJ
Tel: 01527 570444
Website: www.dietaryneedsdirect.co.uk
Suppliers of products for people with food allergies or intolerances or who are on special diets.

Doves Farm Foods Ltd
Salisbury Road
Hungerford
Berkshire RG17 0RF
Tel: 01488 684880
Website: www.dovesfarm.co.uk
Spelt, gram, maize, rice, buckwheat, rye and organic flours; vegan, dairy-free and soya-free digestive biscuits. Range of gluten- and wheat-free products, including biscuits, cookies, cereals and flapjacks.

Dr Hadwen Trust
84A Tilehouse Street
Hitchin
Herts SG5 2DY
Tel: 01462 436819
Website: www.drhadwentrust.org.uk
Large range of handmade adult and children's chocolates, fudge, Turkish delight, Christmas pudding, sweets, truffles – all vegan, milk-free and egg-free. Available by mail order or online.

Ecomil
c/o Organico RealFoods [distributor]
Website: www.ecomil.com
Produces selection of alternative milks, including quinoa drink; almond drink; hazelnut drink; instant almond drink powder; organic almond and soya drink.

Ener-G Foods Inc.
c/o General Dietary Ltd [distributor]
Website: www.ener-g.com
US company producing egg replacer and a wide range of foods free from wheat, gluten, dairy, soya, egg, corn, etc. Rice bread and tapioca bread are especially useful in exclusion diets and for multiple allergies.

Everfresh Natural Foods
Gatehouse Close
Aylesbury
Bucks HP19 3DE
Tel: 01296 425333
Website: www.sunnyvaleorganic.com
Organic bread, cakes and puddings free from yeast, milk, gluten, eggs (and vegan): banana cake, chocolate chip cake, fruit cake, stem ginger cake, lemon cake, etc. Available at healthfood shops and by mail order.

Fabulous Bakin' Boys
Avenue 2
Station Lane
Witney
OX28 4YT
Tel: 01993 777444
Website: www.bakinboys.co.uk
Suppliers of nut-free muffins, cakes and other products all labelled with a bold nut-free symbol. Available from supermarkets and online.

Fayrefield Foods Ltd
Englesea House
Barthomley Road
Crewe
Cheshire CW1 5UF
Tel: 01270 589311
Website: www.fayrefield.com
Suppliers of non-dairy alternatives to ice-cream (Swedish Glace). All products are free from lactose and cholesterol, and contain no genetically modified ingredients.

First Foods
PO Box 140
Amersham
Bucks HP6 6XD
Tel: 01494 431355
Website: www.first-foods.com
Products based on oats free from milk, dairy and soya. Oat milk and ice-creams in a variety of flavours. Available from major retailers and healthfood shops.

Galaxy Nutritional Foods
Website: www.galaxyfoods.com
Dairy-free soya cheese slices – widely available. They also make rice cheese slices but these are not dairy-free as they contain casein.

General Dietary Ltd
PO Box 38
Kingston upon Thames
Surrey KT2 7YP
Tel: 020 8336 2323
Website: www.ener-g.com
Manufacturers of a variety of special diet products, including gluten-free breads and baguettes, rice breads, and pastas, egg replacer, biscuits, xantham gum, cereals, bread and pastry mixes that are free from wheat, soya, maize, gluten, egg, milk, lactose, casein and yeast. Available from any chemist dispensary and most healthfood shops. Associated brand names are Ener-G *and* Tinkyada.

Glutafin
see Nutricia Dietary Care

Gluten Free Foods Ltd
Unit 270 Centennial Park
Centennial Avenue
Elstree
Borehamwood
Herts WD6 3SS
Tel: 020 8953 4444
Website: www.glutenfree-foods.co.uk
Trades under the following names:
Glutano: *gluten- and wheat-free
biscuits, cakes, breads, bread mixes and
pastas; selection of savoury snacks,
pretzels and crackers.* Barkat: *rice
breads, pizza crust, bread mix free from
milk, yeast, gluten, wheat and egg.
Available from supermarkets, healthfood
shops, chemists/pharmacists and by
mail order or online.*

Granovita UK Ltd
5 Stanton Close
Finedon Road Industrial Estate
Wellingborough
Northants NN8 4HN
Tel: 01933 273717
Website: www.granovita.co.uk
*Full range of products suitable for
dairy-free and gluten-free diets; soya
milks;* Soyage *yoghurts in various
flavours. Yeast and vegetable spreads.
Various organic vegetable patés, and
fruit and vegetable juices. Egg-free
mayonnaise. Fruit bars. Many products
are vegan, so suitable for diets free from
dairy, egg and fish. Available at
healthfood shops and some
supermarkets.*

Haldane Foods Group
Howard Way
Newport Pagnall
Bucks MK16 9PY
Tel: 01908 211311
Website: www.haldanefoods.co.uk
*Vegetarian and vegan foods under brand
names* Granose, Realeat, Organic *and*
Direct Foods. *Includes a range of soya
milks, cream, yoghurts, snack pots and
frozen meals in a variety of flavours.
Widely available.*

Humdinger Ltd
Gothenburg Way
Sutton Fields Industrial Estate
Kingston upon Hull HU7 0YG
Tel: 01482 625790
Website: www.humdinger-foods.co.uk
*Suppliers of dairy-free chocolate bars:
original, rice crackle, roasted almond,
tangerine. Available in supermarkets
and healthfood shops.*

Isle of Bute Foods Ltd
Orissor House
Craigmore Road
Rothesay
Isle of Bute PA20 9LB
Tel: 01700 505357
Website: www.scheese.co.uk
*Selection of hard dairy-free cheeses.
Recipes available on the website.*

It's Nut Free Ltd
Moxton Court
Thurston Road
Northallerton DL6 2NG
Tel: 01609 775660
Website: www.itsnutfree.com
*Suppliers of biscuits, cakes, celebration
and wedding cakes, cereals, desserts.
Available from supermarkets or online.*

Juvela
SHS International Ltd
100 Wavertree Boulevard
Wavertree Technology Park
Liverpool L7 9PT
Tel: 0151 228 1992
Website: www.juvela.co.uk
A selection of gluten-free breads, bread mixes, biscuits and crackers, available at pharmacies/chemists and on prescription.

Kallo Foods
Coopers Place
Coombe Lane
Wormley
Godalming
Surrey GU8 5SZ
Tel: 01428 685100
Website: www.kallofoods.com
A selection of gluten-, wheat- and soya-free products.

Karen's Cakes
Tel: 020 8203 8049
Email: krcakes@yahoo.co.uk
Home-baked gluten- and wheat-free cakes; also suitable for vegetarians.

Kealth Foods Ltd
Unit 4
Hirwaun Industrial Estate
Hirwaun
Aberdare CF44 9UP
Tel: 0845 082 2350
Website: www.kealthfoods.com
Selection of allergy-free ready meals delivered to your home. (Also supplied to hospitals and NHS trusts.)

Kinnerton (Confectionery) Co. Ltd
1000 Highgate Studios
53–79 Highgate Road
London NW5 1TL
Tel: 020 7284 9500
Website: www.kinnerton.com
Have separated their factory into nut and nut-free zones, so their nut-free chocolate is guaranteed to be nut-free. Catalogue available for children's novelty bars, Easter eggs and a Christmas selection. Widely available in supermarkets.

Lifestyle Healthcare Ltd
Centenary Business Park
Henley-on-Thames RG9 1DS
Tel: 01491 570000
Website: www.gfdiet.com
A selection of biscuits free from gluten, wheat and milk. Gluten-free breads, fruit buns, rolls, puddings, sweet and savoury pastry goods, all freshly cooked. Available on prescription at pharmacies/chemists. Home deliveries throughout the UK. Allergycare range: egg-free omelette mix, egg replacer, gluten-free stuffing and baking powder. Ultrapharm: selection of gluten- and wheat-free products. Valpiform: selection of everyday and luxury gluten- and wheat-free products. Whizzers: dairy-free confectionery.

Lyme Regis Fine Foods Ltd
Station Industrial Estate
Liphook
Hampshire GU30 7DR
Tel: 01428 722900
Website: www.lymeregisfoods.com
Range of snacks free from wheat, milk and sugar; fruit bars; chocolate- coated marzipan bar. From healthfood shops and supermarkets.

Matthews Foods plc
The Healy Complex
Healy Road
Ossett
West Yorkshire WF5 8NE
Information: 08000 284499
Tel: 01924 272534
Website: www.purespreads.com
Manufacturers of Pure *dairy-free
sunflower spread, soya spread and
organic spread.*

Meridian Foods Ltd
The Estate Office
Sutton Scotney
Hampshire SO21 3JW
Tel: 01962 761935
Website: www.meridianfoods.co.uk
*Available widely in supermarkets,
healthfood shops and online.*

M H Foods
5 Church Trading Estate
Slade Green Road
Slade Green
Erith
Kent DA8 2JA
Tel: 01322 337711
Website: www.parmazano.com
Florentino *Parmazano non-animal
dairy/milk/egg-free Parmesan-style
'cheese'. Widely available.*

Mrs Leeper's Pasta
c/o Granovita UK Ltd
*Corn and rice pastas free from wheat
and gluten.*

Nutricia Dietary Care
Newmarket Avenue
White Horse Business Park
Trowbridge
Wiltshire BA14 0XQ
Tel: 01225 711 801
Websites: www.nutriciadietarycare.co.uk
             www.glutafin.co.uk
*A variety of products free from gluten,
wheat, milk and egg.* Rite Diet: *breads,
rolls, baking powder and flour mixes.*
Glutafin: *large variety of bread, cakes,
mixes, biscuits, pizza bases and
baguettes. Available on prescription at
pharmacies/chemist shops.*

Nutrition Point Ltd
13 Taurus Park
Westbrook
Warrington WA5 5ZT
Tel: 07041 544044
Website: www.nutritionpoint.co.uk
*A large selection of bread, cake, scone
and pastry mixes free from wheat and
gluten from brands* Dietary Specials
and Trufree. *Recipes available on their
website.*

Oatly
c/o Wassen International Ltd
14 The Mole Business Park
Leatherhead
Surrey KT22 7BA
Tel: 01372 379828
Website: www.oatly.com
*Organic dairy and genetically-modified-
free oat-based milk and cream. Available
from supermarkets, healthfood shops
and online*

Ok Foods Ltd
Edenholme Bakery
Lazonby
Penrith
Cumbria CA10 1BG
Tel: 01768 881811
Website: www.ok-foods.co.uk
Selection of guaranteed wheat-, gluten-
and dairy-free products; e.g. fruit
fingers, cake slices, whole cakes and
sponge puddings.

Organico RealFoods Ltd
Unit 3, City Limits
Danehill
Lower Earley
Reading RG6 4UP
Tel: 0118 923 8760
Website: www.organico.homestead.com
Suppliers of a wide range of organic
foods, including Ecomil *alternative*
milks (quinoa, almond, hazelnut, soya).

Orgran
c/o Community Foods [distributor]
Website: www.orgran.com
Whole-egg-replacer and a wide range of
wheat- and gluten-free products,
including pastas, fruit bars, pancake
mix, gravy mix, pizza mix, falafel mix,
corn cakes, rice cakes, crispbreads and
spaghetti in tomato sauce. Available
online and from healthfood shops,
pharmacies/chemists and some
supermarkets.

Pamela's Products Inc
Website: www.pamelasproducts.com
A variety of gluten-free biscuits: pecan
shortbread, butter shortbread, ginger
cookies, shortbread swirl, peanut butter
cookies, lemon shortbread, carob
hazelnut cookies, simply chocolate
shortbread. Available at healthfood
shops.

Plamil Foods
Plamil House
4 Bowles Well Gardens
Dover Road
Folkestone
Kent CT19 6PQ
Tel: 01303 850588
Website: www.plamilfoods.co.uk
Variety of dairy-free chocolates: plain,
milk and flavoured. Carob drops.
Dairy-free milk. Egg-free mayonnaise:
plain, garlic, lemon, tarragon, organic.

Pleniday
c/o Tree of Life UK Ltd
Large range of gluten-free products,
including low-fat varieties. Biscuits
include: chocolate chip crunch, coconut
crunch, ginger nut and sultana spice.
Cakes, crispy bars, muesli-flavoured
mini rice cakes, bread mixes, cake
mixes, pastas. Many lines on
prescription.

Provamel
see Alpro Soya
Website: www.provamel.com

Pure Wine Co.
Ocean House
51 Alcantara Crescent
Ocean Village
Southampton SO14 3HR
Tel: 0844 800 9157
Website: www.purewine.co.uk
*Selection of organic wines that are
vegan (i.e. not clarified with any egg,
milk or fish products). Available by mail
order and to trade.*

R J Foods Ltd
Units 1–5
7 Airfield Road
Airfield Industrial estate
Christchurch
Dorset BH23 3TQ
Tel: 01202 481 471
Website: www.rjfoods-flapjack.com
*Vegan (free from milk, eggs, animal
products) fruit bars and flapjacks;
vegetarian fruit bars, flapjacks and
individually wrapped cookies (some
vegan).*

Rakusen's
Rakusen House
Clayton Wood Rise
Ring Road, West Park
Leeds
W Yorks LS16 6QN
Tel: 0113 278 4821
Website: www.rakusens.co.uk
*No dairy on site. Dairy-free margarine
Tomor. Also a selection of kosher foods
that are dairy-free, including non-dairy
ice-creams. Biscuits, cookies, crackers,
soups. Vegetable and/or soya based.
Widely available. Product-allergy
information sheets also available.*

Redwood Wholefood Company
Redwood House
60 Burkitt Road
Corby NN17 4DT
Tel: 01536 400557
Website: www.redwoodfoods.co.uk
*Large selection of vegan foods, including
the Cheezly selection of alternative
cheeses. All suitable for egg-free and
milk-free diets.*

Rich Products Ltd
Unit 5
Solent Gate
Speedfields Park
Newgate Lane
Fareham PO14 1TL
Tel: 01329 822255
Website: www.richuk.com
*Whip topping 'cream' available from
healthfood and kosher shops.*

Safe to Eat
Calico Lane
Furness Vale SK23 7SW
Tel: 01663 744452
Website: www.safetoeatfood.com
*Sauces and soups made in an
environment guaranteed safe for people
with food allergy. Available online and
in some supermarkets.*

Sauces of Choice Ltd
Unit 5
Lufton Heights Commerce Park
Boundary Way
Yeovil BA22 8UY
Tel: 01935 431924
Website: www.saucesofchoice.co.uk
*Large selection of savoury and sweet
sauces, catering for most special diets.
Available by mail order or online.*

Schär
Imported by Nutrition Point Ltd
Website: www.schaer.com
*A good selection of products free from
wheat and gluten, many of which are
available on prescription. Includes
Schär biscuits, pastas, bread, rolls,
crispbreads, crackers and cakes.*

Scientific Hospital Supplies (SHS)
100 Wavertree Boulevard
Wavertree Technology Park
Liverpool L7 9PT
Tel: 0151 228 8161
Websites:
www.shsweb.co.uk
for whole egg and egg white replacer
www.juvela.co.uk
*for product information
Manufacture the Juvela range of wheat-
free and gluten-free products, many of
which are available on prescription.*

Shepherd Boy Foods
Healthcross House
Cross Street
Syston
Leicester LE7 2JG
Tel: 0116 260 2992
Website: www.shepherdboy.co.uk
*Just So carob bars: crispy, orange,
peppermint, ginger – free from milk, egg
and animal products (vegan). Also fruit,
nut and seed bars; muesli; hemp oil
capsules (similar to cod liver oil; contain
omega 3 and 6).*

SoGood International
Stanley House
57–59 Broadway
City Road
Peterborough PE1 1SY
Customer Careline 0800 328 0423
Website: www.sogood123.com
*SoGood range of soya beverages,
available from most supermarkets and
healthfood stores. Website has product
details and recipes.*

Sojasun
c/o Goodness Direct [distributor]
*Selection of soya-based dairy-free vegan
yoghurts, desserts, milks, available from
healthfood shops and most wholesalers.
Products contain probiotics.*

Soya Health Foods Ltd
1 The Courtyard
Ashley Road
Hale
Cheshire WA14 3NG
Tel: 0161 924 1050
Website: www.soya-group.com
*Sunrise: no-added-sugar soya milk
drinks and powders; dairy-free choc ices.*

Stiletto Foods (UK) Ltd
Fountains Mall
High Street
Odiham RG29 1LP
Tel: 0845 130 0869
*Mrs Crimble's cakes free from egg,
dairy and wheat. Available from
healthfood shops, supermarkets and
distributors.*

Sun Foods
Van Guard Trading Centre
16 Marshgate Lane
London E15 2NH
Tel: 020 8555 7075
*A variety of cakes and breads free from
eggs, gluten, wheat and dairy. Available
from healthfood shops and distributors.*

Traidcraft plc
Kingsway
Gateshead
Tyne & Wear NE11 0NE
Tel: 0191 491 0591
Website: www.traidcraft.co.uk
*Continental dairy-free chocolate.
Available by mail order or through
healthfood stores.*

Tree of Life UK Ltd
Coaldale Road
Lymedale Business Park
Newcastle under Lyme
Staffs ST5 9QX
Tel: 01782 567100
Website: www.treeoflifeuk.com
*Suppliers of a wide range of foods for
people requiring a special diet.*

Triano Brands Ltd
5th floor, Congress House
14 Lyon Road
Harrow
Middx HA1 2FD
Tel: 020 8861 4443
Website: www.trianobrands.co.uk
Snowcrest *'cream' whip.* Tofutti *frozen
desserts and cheese spreads.* Turtle
Mountain *ice-creams.*

Tropical Source
*Dairy-free chocolate made on a
production line 100% dairy-free.
Available from vegan chocolate suppliers
or by special order from healthfood
shops, or online from the US-based
supplier of vegan foods on
www.wellnessgrocer.com*

Trufree
see Nutrition Point

Ultrapharm
Centennial Business Park
Henley-on-Thames
Oxon RG9 1DS
Tel: 01491 570 000
Website: www.gfdiet.com
*Gluten-free bakers with a wide range of
breads, cakes, crackers and biscuits,
available on prescription and by mail
order as* Lifestyle Healthcare. *Also
own* Allergycare – *dairy-free
confectionery; alternative milks; cooking
aids; gluten-free gravy powder, baking
powder and stuffing mix. Whole-egg
replacer.*

Vance's Darifree
Website: www.darifree.co.uk
*Potato milk powder in original and
chocolate flavours. This is a US
company; see the website for details
of UK stockists.*

Village Bakery
Melmerby
Penrith
Cumbria CA10 1HE
Tel: 01768 881 811
Website: www.village-bakery.com
Special diet products on mail order,
including products free from wheat,
yeast, dairy, sugar and salt. Bread,
biscuits and cakes. Selection of
Christmas products suitable for wheat-
and gluten-free diets. Also a good
selection of vegan cakes, biscuits and
slices. Has a dedicated production line
for products free from dairy, gluten
and wheat.Available by mail order
or through selected stockists (list of
stockists available).

Vintage Roots Ltd
Farley Farms/Bridge Farm
Reading Road
Arborfield
Berks RG2 9HT
Tel: 0800 980 4992
Website: www.vintageroots.co.uk
Vegan, organic and low-sulphur wines,
spirits and beers, available by mail order
or at selected healthfood shops and
specialist off-licences.

Vitaquell
Various dairy-free margarines available
in supermarkets and healthfood shops.

Vitariz
c/o Suma [distributors]
Organic rice drink made in Italy and
distributed via the wholesalers.
Available direct from the wholesaler or
from healthfood shops.

Viva!
8 York Court
Wilder Street
Bristol BS2 8QH
Tel: 0117 944 1000
Website: www.viva.org.uk
Vegan organisation selling dairy-free
fudge, chocolate beans and chocolate in
bars and boxes. Available only by mail
order. Also a good selection of vegan
cookery books.

Whole Earth Foods Ltd
2 Valentine Place
London SE1 8QH
Tel: 020 7633 5900
Variety of organic dairy-free, gluten-free
cereals and chocolate (chocolate under
the name Green & Black's*). You should*
read the individual product labels to
check for their suitability for your diet;
not all their chocolate is dairy-free. Free
recipe booklet on request. Widely
available, and via mail order.

SPECIALIST INFANT FORMULAS

Cow & Gate and Milupa
White Horse Business Park
New Market Avenue
Trowbridge
Wiltshire BA14 0XQ
Tel: 01225 768 381
Helpline: 08457 623623/4
Websites:
Cow & Gate: www.cowandgate.co.uk
for healthcare professionals:
Milupa: www.milupa-aptamil.co.uk
for healthcare professionals:
www.milupap-aptamil.co.uk
Cow & Gate products: Pepti *(whey
hydrolysate without MCT);* Pepti-
Junior *(whey hydrolysates with MCT);*
Infasoy *(soya formula)*
Milupa product: Prejomin *(pork & soya
formula)*

Farley's and Heinz
H J Heinz Co Ltd
6 South Building
Hayes Park
Hayes
Middx UB4 8AL
Tel: 0800 528 5757
Tinytums Careline: 0800 212 991
Farley's Careline: 0845 057 0057
Website: www.heinz.co.uk
Websites: www.tinytums.co.uk
            www.farleyscloserbynature.co.uk
Products: Farley's *soya formula*

Mead Johnson Nutritionals
Uxbridge Business Park
Sanderson Road
Uxbridge UB8 1DH
Tel: 00800 8834 2568
Website: www.meadjohnson.com
Producers of Nutramigen,
Nutramigen 2, Prejestimil, Prosobee

Nestlé Nutrition
St George's House
Wellesley Road
Croydon
Surrey CR9 1NR
Tel: 020 8667 6335
Website:
www.nestle.co.uk/nutrition/infantnutrition
Products: NAN H.A.1 *and* NAN H.A.2
*– partially hydrolysed formula for
allergy prevention (not suitable for
treatment/management of food allergy).*

SHS International Ltd
100 Wavertree Boulevard
Wavertree Technology Park
Liverpool L7 9PT
Tel: 0151 228 8161
Website: www.shsweb.co.uk
Products: Neocate *(elemental formula);*
Pepdite *(hydrolysed pork and soya
amino acid formula);* Pepdite 1+
*(hydrolysed pork and soya amino acid
formula for infants 1 year plus);*
NeocateAdvance *(child amino acid
formula).*

SMA Nutrition
Huntercombe Lane South
Taplow
Maidenhead
Berks SL6 0PH
Careline: 0845 776 2900
Website: www.smanutrition.co.uk
*Make a variety of formula and specialist
milks, including SMA Wysoy (soya
formula). Available on prescription and
over the counter.*

DISTRIBUTORS OF SPECIAL DIET PRODUCTS
(also called wholesalers or suppliers)

AllergyFree Direct
'Conna-Mara'
Maer Down Road
Bude
Cornwall EX23 8NG
Tel: 01288 356396
Website: www.allergyfreedirect.com
Mail order specialist for foods free from wheat, gluten, milk and egg; vegan and vegetarian foods also available. The website is easy to navigate with the categories clearly labelled and giving the ingredients used for each product. It also contains a glossary.

Community Foods
Micross
Brent Terrace
London NW2 1LT
Tel: 020 8450 9419
Website: www.communityfoods.co.uk
Distributor of Orgran *products.*

Goodness Direct
South March
Daventry
Northants NN11 4PH
Tel: 0871 871 6611
Textphone: 07973 326996
Website: goodnessdirect.co.uk
Supplier of thousands of special diet products, including frozen items, by phone, mail order or online. Next day delivery. Catalogue available.

Infinity Foods Co-operative Ltd
67 Norway Street
Portslade
E Sussex BN41 1AE
Tel: 01273 424060
Website: www.infinityfoods.co.uk
Organic food wholesaler and distributor selling products suitable for all special diets.

Marigold Healthfoods Ltd
102 Camley Street
London NW1 0PF
Tel: 020 7388 4515
Website: www.marigoldhealth.com
Distributor for Engevita *nutritional yeast flakes that can be used as a cheese substitute to sprinkle on pizza, pasta, etc., and a variety of bouillon powders that are suitable for diets free from yeast, wheat, gluten, soya, egg and cow's milk. Many other lines also available.*

Suma Wholefoods
Lacy Way
Lowfields Business Park
Elland
W Yorkshire HX5 9DB
Tel: 0845 458 2290
Website: www.suma.co.uk
A distributor of other companies' products but also has its own brands. All are vegetarian; some are vegan and organic. A range of dairy-free and soya-free full-fat and low-fat spreads. Vegannaise: egg-free mayonnaise. Some soups are free from gluten, milk, egg and soya; dairy-free pesto; and much, much more.

Windmill Organics
34a Clifton Road
Kingston upon Thames
Surrey KT2 6PH
Tel: 020 8547 2775
Website: www.windmillorganics.com
Wholesaler for organic foods, including many that are suitable for special diets. Biona Foods for wheat- and gluten-free cookies, cakes, pastas, breads, mixes. Vegan spreads free from dairy and soya.

SUPERMARKETS AND STORES

Asda
Customer Services Department
Asda House
Great Wilson Street
Leeds LS11 5AD
Tel: 0500 10 00 55
Website: www.asda.co.uk
'Free from' booklets available on request.

Co-op (CWS) Ltd
Customer Services
CWS Ltd
Freepost MR9 473
Manchester M4 8BA
Tel: 0800 0686 727
Textphone: 0800 0686 717
Website: www.co-op.co.uk
Will provide, on request, 'free from' lists free of charge for their own-brand products.

Marks and Spencer
Retail Customer Services
Chester Business Park
Wrexham Road
Chester CH4 9GA
Tel: 0845 302 1234
Website: www.marksandspencer.com
Will provide, on request, information on own-brand foods that are suitable for special diets.

Morrisons
Customer Services
Hillmore House
Gain Lane
Bradford BD3 7DL
Tel: 0845 611 6111
Website: www.morrisons.co.uk
'Free from' lists for various special diets available on request.

J Sainsbury plc
Customer Services
33 Holborn
London EC1N 2HT
Tel: 0800 636262
Website: www.sainsbury.co.uk
'Free from' lists for various special diets available on request. Also has own-brand free-from products.

Somerfield Stores Ltd
Customer Relations
Somerfield House
Hawkfield Business Park
Whitchurch Lane
Bristol BS14 0TJ
Tel: 0117 935 9359
Website: www.somerfield.co.uk
'Free from' lists for various special diets available on request.

Tesco
Nutrition Advice Service
PO Box 73
Dryburgh Industrial Estate
Baird Avenue
Dundee DD1 9NF
Tel: 0800 505 555
Website: www.tesco.co.uk
'Free from' lists for various special diets available on request. Also has own-brand free-from products.

Waitrose
Nutrition Advice Service
Doncastle Road
Bracknell
Berkshire RG12 8YA
Tel: 0800 188 884
Website: www.waitrose.co.uk
'Free from' lists for various special diets available on request.

Appendix 2
Useful Websites

INFORMATION

Most of the organisations listed in Appendix 1 have a website. Below are given websites not generally listed in Appendix 1. Please note that these are given for your information only and should *not* be used to replace professional advice and treatment. Remember, too, that websites outside the UK will often use different terminology, weights and measures, trade names.

www.allallergy.net
Huge website created with the aim of pulling together all the other websites related to allergy

www.allergicchild.com
A website created by parents of an allergic child. It aims to provide understanding and information as well as links to other websites and book information

www.allergies.about.com
All about allergies, in user-friendly language

www.allergyaction.org
Very helpful site that includes translations, food lists, advice and presentations on aspects of severe food allergy; has extremely useful information for people with allergies and their families and healthcare professionals, and caterers.
Has also produced a DVD and training pack on allergy awareness for food handlers. See www.allergytraining.com or call 01727 866779

www.allergyinschools.org.uk
Brilliant information for parents, nurseries, pre-schools and schools, from the Anaphylaxis Campaign

www.allergypack.com
Supplier of the Pen Pal, which is a versatile carry-bag for the EpiPen. The case is detachable from the strap and has Velcro straps for hooking onto bike handles etc., is insulated and shock resistant

www.allergytraining.com
Site packed with advice, catering information and lots more; developed by Hazel Gowland, Food Adviser to the Anaphylaxis Campaign

www.anaphylaxis.org
Canadian equivalent of the UK Anaphylaxis Campaign

www.angelfire.com/mi/FAST
A non-commercial US site, run by people with a food allergy, devoted to educating the public about food allergy, with on-line discussion, support groups etc.

www.baronmoss.demon.co.uk
The website of Helen Stephenson, who has several food intolerances, including dairy products and eggs. Has excellent links to websites related to food allergies

www.cateringforallergy.org
For the catering industry with information and advice about catering for people with severe food allergies (from the Anaphylaxis Campaign)

www.choclat.com
Chocolate emporium: pareve speciality chocolates and other kosher confections for people needing dairy-free sweets

www.dairyfree.org.uk
Information about dairy-free products, links, questions and forums

www.dsftp.dial.pipex.com
A site devoted to dairy allergy and intolerance. Information, resources, articles and general help. Very informative

www.epipen.co.uk
All about the EpiPen

www.foodallergy.org
Website of the Food Allergy and Anaphylaxis Network (a non-profit-making US organisation), devoted to educating the public about food allergy and anaphylaxis, and advancing research. It publishes six newsletters a year and offers a range of resources

www.foodsmatter.com
A site built around an archive of articles that have appeared in the Foods Matter *magazine. It covers food allergy and other conditions such as asthma, eczema, coeliac disease, arthritis and ME*

www.harid.co.uk
Lists restaurants and hotels that cater for special diets

www.inside-story.com
Useful website with information on many aspects of allergy (including anaphylaxis), recipes, book list and links to related sites

www.milkfree.org
An informative parent-run site about the dairy-allergic child

www.NoMilk.com
Information, recipes and advice for people with lactose maldigestion, milk allergy and casein intolerance

www.non-dairy.org
Comprehensive and informative site run by parents of children with allergy to dairy foods

www.peanutallergy.com
US site devoted to all aspects of peanut allergy

www.protectube.com
Provide protective tubes for EpiPen. They are waterproof and buoyant, UV-protected and very durable. No more broken tubes or lost tops! Also carrying cases (Epi-Tote and Epi-Tote Twin) for the tubes

www.specialdietsconsulting.co.uk
Online support organisation for people with food allergy/intolerance, and for the catering and restaurant industry.

www.veg.org/veg
Independent, definitive internet guide for vegetarians and vegans, with many valuable resources, recipes and links to related sites

www.veganvillage.co.uk
An excellent site with information on everything vegan

www.veggieheaven.com
The site to find vegetarian and vegan recipes, UK restaurant guide, nutritional guide, glossary, useful tips and links to related sites

www.zoniinc.com
Sales only. The Epi-belt will protect your emergency auto-injector in many conditions and, because you wear it, it provides quick easy access if required. Available as a single or double case attached to a belt or as a single or double holster

BOOKS

The websites listed below (not mentioned elsewhere) give details of and/or produce information books and recipe books for allergy

www.amazon.com and **www.amazon.co.uk**
On-line booksellers with a good range of recipe books and books on food allergy and intolerance and special diets

www.hallPublications.com
Books and other publications on food allergy and intolerance

Appendix 3
Useful Publications

Below are listed publications that you might find helpful. In some cases they are published outside the UK but are available through your bookshop or local library or via the internet. Websites that have information about useful books are listed in Appendix 2.

INFORMATION BOOKS
Berlitz European Menu Reader. Berlitz Publishing, London, 2003.

Bird K, Farhall R, Rofe A, Whitlock J (Editors). *Animal-free Shopper*, 7th edition. Vegan Society, St Leonards on Sea, E Sussex, 2005 [directory of animal-, dairy-, egg-free products from food to cosmetics and cleaning agents]

Clough J. *Allergies – answers at your fingertips*, 2nd edition. Class Publishing, London, 2007

Collins L. *Caring for Your Child with Severe Food Allergies: emotional support and practical advice from a parent who's been there*. Wiley, Chichester, 1999

Durham SR. *ABC of Allergies*. BMJ Books, London, 1998

Joneja JV. *Dietary Management of Food Allergies and Intolerances: a comprehensive guide*, 2nd edn. J A Hall Publications, Burnaby BC, Canada, 1999 [also available from Merton Books]

Marienhoff Coss L. *How to Manage Your Child's Life-threatening Food Allergies*. Plumtree Press, Lake Forest, CA, 2004

The Really Jewish Food Guide. London Beth Din 2005, London, 2005

Sicherer SH. *The Complete Peanut Allergy Handbook*. Penguin, London, 2005

Williams D, Williams A, Croker L. *Life-threatening Allergic Reactions: understanding and coping with anaphylaxis*. Piatkus, London, 1997

EATING OUT AND HOLIDAY ACCOMMODATION
Berlitz European Menu Reader. Berlitz Publishing, London, 2003

Bourke A (Editor) *Vegetarian Europe*. Vegetarian Guides, London

Bourke A, Gaynor P. *Vegetarian London*. Cruelty Free Living Publisher

Bourke A, Todd A. *Vegetarian Britain*, Vegetarian Guides, London

Bourke A, Todd A. *Vegetarian France*, Vegetarian Guides, London

Collin SM. *Eating Out in Five Languages*. Bloomsbury, London, 2004

Rodger G. (Editor). *Vegan Passport*. Vegan Society, St Leonards on Sea, E Sussex, 2002 [what vegans eat and don't eat, in 38 languages – useful for allergy to meat, fish, shellfish, milk, egg]

Vegan Society. *Vegan Travel Guide*. Vegan Society, St Leonards on Sea, E Sussex, [contains information on suitable places to stay and eat for vegans and those on egg-free, milk-free, fish/shellfish-free and meat-free diets, as well as details on hotels, B&Bs, guest houses, restaurants, cafés and tearooms, take-aways, pubs, wine bars and speciality holidays in Britain] Available from your local bookshop or direct from Vegetarian Guides Ltd, PO Box 2284, London W1A 5UH (www.vegetarianguides.co.uk)

Weitzel AM. *Vegetarian Visitor: where to eat and stay in Britain*. Jon Carpenter Publishing, Chipping Norton, Oxon, 2006 [lists 300 establishments, many of which are used to catering for special diets]

CHILDREN'S BOOKS

Alexander the Elephant who couldn't eat Peanuts. Available from Allergy Essentials (59A Robertson Road, suite 148, Nepean Ontario, Ontario K2H 5Y9, Canada)

Allie the Allergic Elephant. Available from Jungle Communications Inc. , 2002 (Suite 3002500 North Circle Drive, Colorado Springs, CO 80919, USA), or from your local bookshop or via the internet if you quote the ISBN 1–58628–050–3

Cyril the Squirrel. Anaphylaxis Campaign, Farnborough, Hants, 1996 [about a squirrel who is allergic to nuts, the story is designed to help children come to terms with nut allergy]

Pre-schooler's Guide to Peanut Allergy. Ticketar Company, Vancouver BC V5N 2E4, Canada (www.mcd.on.ca/ticketar/)

Troon H. *Aaron's Awful Allergies*. Kids Can Press, Toronto, Ontario, Canada, and Buffalo, NY, 1998.

Ureel J. *The Peanut Pickle*. First Page Publications, Livonia, MI, 2004

Weiner E. *Taking Food Allergies to School* (Special kids in school). Jayjo Books, Plainview, NY, 1999

Young MC. *The Peanut Allergy Answer Book*. Fair Winds Press, Gloucester, MA, 2001

Zevy A. *No Nuts for Me*. Tumbleweed Press, 1999 (Unit 11, 401 Magnetic Drive, Downsview, Ontario M3J 3H9, Canada) [a story about how a little boy handles his food allergy at school]

RECIPE BOOKS

Berriedale-Johnson M. *The Everyday Wheat- and Gluten-free Cookbook*, Grub Street, London, 1998

Berriedale-Johnson M. *Allergy-Aware Schools Catering Manual*, Berrydales Books, London, 2005

Bronfman D, Bronfman R. *Calciyum! Delicious calcium-rich dairy-free vegetarian recipes*. Bromedia, Toronto, Ontario, 1998

Cole C. L. *Not Milk . . . Nut Milks*. Woodbridge Press, Santa Barbara, CA, 1997

Crosthwaite F. *How to Eat Well again on a Wheat, Gluten and Dairy Free Diet.** Merton Books, Twickenham, 1997

Dumke NM. *Easy Bread Making for Special Diets.* Adapt Books, Louisville, CO, 1998

Emro R. *Bakin' Without Eggs.* St Martins Griffin, New York, 1999

Fenster C. *Special Diet Celebrations – no wheat, gluten, dairy or eggs.* Savory Palate Inc., Littleton, CO, 1999

Graimes N. *The Vegan Cookbook.* Lorenz Books, London, 2000

Greer R. *Easy Wheat, Milk and Egg-free Cooking.* Thorsons, London, 2001

Hall PH. *101 Fabulous Dairy-free Desserts Everyone Will Love.* Station Hill Openings, Barrytown, NY, 1998

Kidder B. *The Milk-Free Kitchen.* Owl Books, New York, 1991

Lanza L, Morton L. *Totally Dairy-free Cooking.* William Morrow, New York, 1999

McCarty M. *Sweet and Natural: more than 120 naturally sweet and dairy-free desserts.* St Martin's Press, New York, 1999

Pannell M. *The Dairy-Free Cook Book.* Lorenz Books, London, 1999

Rawcliffe P, Ralph R. *The Gluten-free Diet.* Vermilion, London, 1997

Robertson R. *366 Simply Delicious Dairy-free Recipes.* Penguin, London, 1997

Stepaniak J. *The Uncheese Cookbook: creating amazing dairy-free substitutes and classic 'uncheese' dishes.* Book Publishing Co., Summertown, TN, 1994

Wellington CM. *Eating Well Milk-free.* Redpine Distributors, Astorville, Ontario, Canada

Wells D. *What Can I give Him Today?** Merton Books, Twickenham, 1998

Wright T. *Allergy-Free Food.* Hamlyn, London, 2005

Zukin J. *Dairy-Free Cookbook.* Prima Health, Rocklin, CA, 1998

Zukin J. *Raising Your Child Without Milk: reassuring advice and recipes for parents of lactose-intolerant and milk-allergic children.* Prima Publishing, Rocklin, CA, 1995.

* Details of these and other allergy recipe books are available from Action Against Allergy (AAA)

LEAFLETS
Useful leaflets are available from the head offices of most food manufacturers and retailers (supermarkets) and the health promotion department of your local health authority, as well as from the following (contact details in the 'Useful addresses' appendix):

Action Against Allergy
Allergy UK
Anaphylaxis Campaign
Coeliac UK

BOOKLETS

Anaphylaxis and Schools: How we can make it work. Anaphylaxis Campaign, Farnborough*, 2005

Letting Go – teaching an allergic child responsibility. Anaphylaxis Campaign, Farnborough*

Managing Food Allergy. Anaphylaxis Campaign, Farnborough, 2004

Nut Allergy: it's not a game of chance. Anaphylaxis Campaign, Fleet, Hants, 1999 [aimed specifically at young people]

Preston M. *The L-Plate Vegan.* Viva!, Brighton, 2005 [excellent product information on foods free from dairy, eggs, animals]

Preston M. *Managing Food Allergy.* Anaphylaxis Campaign, Farnborough*, 2005

MAGAZINES

Foods Matter a monthly subscription magazine supporting anyone with any kind of restricted diet, no matter what the cause

REPORTS

Committee on Toxicity of Chemicals in Foods, Consumer Products and the Environment, for the Department of Health. *Peanut Allergy.* Department of Health, London, 1998

Department for Education and Skills. *Managing Medicines in Schools and Early Years Settings.* DfES, London, 2005

Department of Health. *A Review of Services for Allergy.* DOH, London, 2006

Royal College of Physicians. *Allergy: the unmet need. A blueprint for better patient care.* RCP, London, 2003

VIDEOS/DVDs

Action for Anaphylaxis Role-play of a child having an anaphylactic reaction at school and the action taken based on training received by the school staff. Anaphylaxis Campaign, Farnborough*

Allergy Awareness training pack with DVD for food handlers – Stage 1 23-minute film with key learning points, tutor's notes and student cards. Explains food allergies, intolerance and coeliac disease; identifies key food allergens and highlights typical risks and how they may be controlled; dramatisation of allergic reaction in a restaurant and emergency treatment. [Awarded a Certificate of Quality and Merit from the Royal Institute of Public Health. Best New Product 2006 – Society of Food Hygiene and Technology] www.allergytraining.com.

The New Kid a video for children with food allergy. Anaphylaxis Campaign. Farnborough*

*Contact details in Appendix 1

Index

Have you found *Food Allergies: Enjoying Life with a Severe Food Allergy* useful and practical? If so, you may be interested in other books from Class Publishing.

Allergies:
Answers at your fingertips'   £17.99
Dr Joanne Clough
A fully updated edition that gives you clear and concise information on allergies – what they are, how they develop and, most importantly, how to deal with them. This authoritative handbook covers a broad range of allergies including asthma, eczema, dermatitis, hayfever, food allergies and anaphylaxis.

> *'Excellent first-hand guidance.'*
> Professor Stephen Holgate,
> Southampton General Hospital

Irritable Bowel Syndrome:
Answers at your fingertips   £17.99
Dr Udi Shmueli
IBS is a trying problem that can affect confidence and lifestyles. It is also remarkably common. All too often, relief at doctors finding 'nothing wrong' is tempered by frustration at the lack of solutions available.

This practical and reassuring book looks at the science behind the symptoms, examines possible ways of finding relief, and gives practical advice on taking control of your condition rather than letting it control you.

Migraine and Other Headaches:
Answers at your fingertips   £14.99
Dr Manuela Fontebasso
Written by an experienced GP with a special interest in headache and migraine, this book acknowledges the uniqueness of every sufferer's experience. Communication between patient and professional is crucial if this complex condition is to be addressed and the best treatment prescribed.

Reading this book will help you understand the nature of your headache, and will give you the confidence to be involved in all areas of decision making.

Asthma:
Answers at your fingertips   £17.99
Dr Mark Levy, Trisha Weller
and Professor Sean Hilton
This book contains over 250 real questions from people with asthma and their families – answered by three medical experts. It contains up-to-date, medically accurate and practical advice on living with asthma.

> *'A helpful and clearly written book.'*
> Dr Martyn Partridge,
> Chief Medical Adviser,
> National Asthma Campaign

Eczema:
Answers at your fingertips   £14.99
Dr Tim Mitchell and Alison Hepplewhite
With answers to hundreds of questions on every aspect of living with eczema, this book will help you find ways to manage your own eczema – or that of your child – to fit in with everyday interests and activities.

> *'What a joy to have a new book which is medically accurate, wide ranging and practical in its approach.'*
> Margaret Cox, Chief Executive,
> National Eczema Society

Beating Depression   £17.99
Dr Stefan Cembrowicz
and Dr Dorcas Kingham
Depression is one of most common illnesses in the world – affecting up to one in four people at some time in their lives. *Beating Depression* shows sufferers and their families that they are not alone, and offers tried and tested techniques for overcoming depression.

> *'All you need to know about depression, presented in a clear, concise and readable way.'*
> Ann Dawson,
> World Health Organization

PRIORITY ORDER FORM

Cut out or photocopy this form and send it (post free in the UK) to:

Class Publishing Priority Service,
FREEPOST 16705
Macmillan Distribution
Basingstoke, RG 21 6ZZ

Tel: 01256 302 699
Fax: 01256 812 558

Please send me urgently
(*tick below*)

Post included
price per copy (*UK only*)

☐ Food Allergies – Enjoying life with a severe food allergy £20.99
(ISBN 13: 978159591468/ISBN 10: 1859591469)

☐ Allergies: Answers at your fingertips £20.99
(ISBN 13: 978159591475/ISBN 10: 1859591477)

☐ Irritable Bowel Syndrome: Answers at your fingertips £20.99
(ISBN 13: 9781859591567/ISBN 10: 1859591566)

☐ Migraine and other headaches: Answers at your fingertips £17.99
(ISBN 13: 9781859591499/ISBN 10: 1859591493)

☐ Asthma: Answers at your fingertips £20.99
(ISBN 13: 9781859591116/ISBN 10: 185959 1116)

☐ Eczema: Answers at your fingertips £17.99
(ISBN 13: 9781859591253/ISBN 10: 1859591256)

☐ Beating Depression £20.99
(ISBN 13: 9781859591505 /ISBN 10: 1859591507)

TOTAL _____

Easy ways to pay

Cheque: I enclose a cheque payable to Class Publishing for _____

Credit card: Please debit my ☐ Mastercard ☐ Visa ☐ Amex

Number .... Expiry date ....

Name ....

My address for delivery is ....

Town .... County .... Postcode ....

Telephone number (*in case of query*) ....

Credit card billing address if different from above ....

Town .... County .... Postcode ....

Class Publishing's guarantee: remember that if, for any reason, you are not satisfied with these books, we will refund all your money, without any questions asked. Prices and VAT rates may be altered for reasons beyond our control.